Support Systems and Community Mental Health

Support Systems and Community Mental Health

Lectures on Concept Development

Gerald Caplan, M.D.

Behavioral Publications New York 1974

Library of Congress Catalog Number 73-12398
ISBN: 0-87705-119-4
Copyright © 1974 by Behavioral Publications

BEHAVIORAL PUBLICATIONS,
72 Fifth Avenue, New York, New York 10011

Printed in the United States of America
This printing 10 9 8 7 6 5 4 3 2 1

Library of Congress Cataloging in Publication Data
Caplan, Gerald.
    Support systems and community mental health.

    1. Community mental health services—Addresses, essays, lectures.
2. Crisis intervention (Psychiatry)—Addresses, essays, lectures.
3. Social psychiatry—Addresses, essays, lectures. I. Title. [DNLM:
1. Community mental health services—Essays. 2. Models,
Psychological—Essays. 3. Psychiatry, Community—Essays. WM9
C244s 1973]
RJ111.C33   362.2′2   73-12398

Contents

Introduction and Overview

This book represents a collection of the concepts I have developed over a period of twenty years, during which time much thought was devoted to the problems inherent in raising the level of mental health in populations. I have been in search of models that will guide me in formulating and organizing programs for the prevention and control of mental disorders. The book consists of selected lectures, delivered by invitation to professional audiences, most of which have not previously been published. Apart from minor copy-editing, I have not altered the original texts, and so readers may study for themselves how my ideas have evolved over the years.

The book begins with a presentation of my latest conceptual model, that of support systems, which I feel represents a significant advance in my thinking. The central concept focuses not so much on the etiology of mental disorders in populations, which is an avenue I have often explored in the past, but on the health-promoting forces at the person-to-person and social levels which enable people to master the challenges and strains of their lives. This new point of view is, as usual, *not* entirely new. Others have dealt with it, and I too have often moved toward it, especially when I have wrestled with the issue of preventing mental disorder by helping people to deal constructively with crises, and when I have tried to understand how social institutions can be modified through planning or consultation in order to provide a salubrious climate for their staffs and clients.

For me this concept never "clicked" until recently; now that it has come into clear focus, I suddenly see a valuable new dimension in many of my earlier conceptual patternings. The purpose of this book is to present the new ideas in their formative stages to my colleagues, along with a short recapitulation of my earlier work, so that they may share some of my excitement at the conceptual development and so that some of them may be stimulated to contribute their own thinking and to mold their own research toward a wider and deeper exploration of this approach.

Chapter II, a lecture first delivered in 1954, represents an early formulation of the public health model applied to community mental health. I focused on the methods to be used by a psychiatrist who accepts the challenge of catering to a total population. My first idea was that in order to affect the lives of the large number of people involved, the psychiatrist must devote much of his effort to consulting with legislators and administrators so as to enable them to develop policies and programs for improving the quality of life, for reducing stress, and for providing services to help people deal with unavoidable predicaments. This led to my formulation of a concept of crisis and of crisis intervention on a widespread scale through the intermediation of existing community "caretaking agents," such as public health nurses and other health workers.

My third idea was that community mental health specialists should also devote effort to direct intervention in the life of families in order to detect and remedy disorders in interpersonal relationships and to foster the development of a health-promoting family milieu that would support the family members in grappling with crises. I based this idea on my earlier research on the identification and treatment of disordered mother-child relationships in Jerusalem well-baby clinics. This lecture demonstrated a movement in my thinking from a focus on the simple linear cause-and-effect sequence in which a pathogenic "carrier-type" mother distorted the personality development of her infant to a more complicated transactional view of a melange of harmful forces inside a family network that might be modified during the upset of a crisis period.

Next I briefly described my research on family crisis, mainly a Harvard study of reactions to the birth of a premature baby; from this I developed ideas about the problems posed for professional caregivers in helping families to deal constructively with the cognitive burdens and emotional upsets of crises. I pointed out that in the same way that families might get upset while helping their members cope with crisis, professional caregivers might themselves become upset while they were supporting the families. I also worked toward implementing a system whereby the community mental health specialist would "backstop" the caregivers through consultation, thereby helping them master their own upsets in this situation. This was an early formulation of what I would later call "theme-interference-reduction," that is, consultation to a caregiver to remedy ineffectiveness in his intervention work with clients, caused by the incursion of subjective distortions triggered by the emotionally hot situation of the crisis.

In the light of the support systems outlined in Chapter I, hindsight reveals that in 1954 I was struggling with a not-clearly-understood formulation of the importance of support for the supporters as a way of dealing with the interpenetration of upset in the successive levels of a supportive system caused by disequilibrium of one of the subsystems.

Chapter III approaches the concept of crisis from another vantage point. In discussing the problem of preventing mental disorder in children by means of early diagnosis and therapy, I examined and discarded as of little value the natural-history-of-disease approach of identifying emotional illness in its earliest stages from characteristic signs and symptoms and then nipping it in the bud by a short intervention. This analysis led me to the more complicated family crisis formulation, and to ideas on the nature and types of crisis that were emerging at that period from our Harvard studies, as illustrated by an analysis of the reactions of a family to the illness and hospitalization of the mother. I showed how the family defended itself against the burdens of the crisis by scapegoating one of the children, who in turn reacted by behavioral upset that aggravated the situation. As the crisis process unfolded, the need to scapegoat the child disappeared, and he was then given the nurturance and support he needed to master his own burdens in coping with his mother's illness. A benign spiral replaced the previous vicious circle that might otherwise have led to an emotional disorder or disturbance of personality development in the child. Once again, I was groping toward the realization that adults as well as children, helpers as well as the helped, are likely to need bolstering during the disequilibrium of crisis, and if this underpinning is not available, mutual weakening may be the result.

In Chapter IV I returned to the concept of pathogenic agents or "carriers" of mental disorder—key persons whose disordered relationships might have a noxious effect on their dependents, particularly during crisis periods of increased susceptibility to interpersonal influence. I chose mothers of infants as my paradigm of such a potentially pathogenic key person, and I described how a disordered mother-child relationship might originate during pregnancy. I then discussed ideas that I had developed during the period 1949-1952 in my Jerusalem well-baby clinic research, and during the following two years at the Harvard Family Health Clinic of the Boston Lying-In Hospital, of using the pregnant woman's increased susceptibility to interpersonal influence as an opportunity to undo the distortions in her relationship to her future infant in their formative stages.

This lecture represented one of my early attempts to capitalize on the leverage possibilities of a crisis disequilibrium, and to recommend that maternity nurses, as the professional caregivers normally in contact with expectant mothers, add a mental hygiene dimension to their regular functions.

In relation to the dominant theme of this book, it is of interest that as far back as 1953 I was emphasizing that, in addition to anticipatory guidance and crisis intervention directly with the pregnant woman, the nurse should devote special effort to mobilizing family and extra-family sources of love and support. I felt that among health professionals nurses were particularly well suited to stimulate such support and to act as bridges of communication and as mediators between their patients and other professional and nonprofessional agencies. I also emphasized that in fulfilling such a function, nurses themselves would need support; I recommended that programs calling upon them to occupy a mental hygiene role should offer the nurses adequate training, supervision, and consultation to provide them with the necessary cognitive and emotional supplies.

In the next chapter, Chapter V, I dealt with the opportunities that the crisis model presented to social workers to contribute to the prevention of mental disorders. Once again, I approached my subject from a different vantage point, allowing me to throw additional light on my thesis.

I formulated an ecological theory of emotional health and disease, and I discussed the complex interplay of the many forces usually at work and our need to shift our preventive focus from the individual patient to the population. I discussed crisis in an individual or family as a special case of system disequilibrium that potentially involved successive levels of the social environment. I advocated that social workers should actually go out into the environment of their clients to investigate these forces on the spot, instead of sitting in their offices listening to reports about them, which had become the customary practice in 1955 when I delivered that lecture.

I then suggested that social workers should share with other mental health specialists the role of mental health consultants to caregiving professionals who were encountering cognitive and emotional difficulties in supporting individuals and families in crisis. And I offered some preliminary formulations of the methods and techniques that they might employ, especially in dealing with the consultation problem that was increasingly arousing my interest in those years—the entanglement of the personal and psychological complications of the caregiver with those of the client he was trying to help. I discussed this in relation to my experience with school teachers and their students, where I had often encountered subjectively derived distortions of the professional relationship which were similar to the disturbances of mother-infant relationships I had studied in well-baby and prenatal clinics. In both cases, I likened the harmful effect to the pathogenicity of a "carrier" of a physical disease, such as typhoid.

In this lecture, I recommended that social worker consultants should avoid tampering with the defensive displacement being used by the caregiving professional in working out his personal problem vicariously by his involvement in the case of his client, and that instead they should utilize their realization of the privately meaningful aspects of the case to exert leverage in the professional sphere. They should protect the formal boundary between the private and professional aspects of the caregiver's life and catalyse a personally meaningful, corrective emotional experience by helping the caregiver master in his client a problem to which he was himself sensitive. This was an early attempt to formulate a consultation method that I did not fully develop until fifteen years later in *The Theory and Practice of Mental Health Consultation*. Its particular significance in our present context is that I was calling on social workers to develop methods of supporting caregivers, and in this connection my lecture advocated that the social worker should also take on the role of mobilizing and maintaining the supportive structure inside the health agency of which she is a staff member, based upon my emphasis that this might be especially necessary during periods of institutional stress.

Chapter VI represents my attempt to recruit an additional caregiver, the family physician, in my campaign of mobilizing a supportive network of community professionals to help people in crisis. I include the paper in this book because it provides a good example of my increasing sophistication in the use of the crisis model as further research provided me with concrete examples of how an understanding of the expectable phenomena of different types of crises could help us work out effective methods of anticipatory guidance and preventive intervention. The paper also formulated the concept of the usual psychological needs of individuals and of social and cultural provisions to satisfy them. It discussed the family as a supportive group, one of whose basic functions is the satisfaction of the psychological needs of its members, both their continuing needs and their specially intense needs for guidance and emotional support in times of acute stress.

Within the framework of this model I emphasized the importance of the role of the family physician in monitoring and promoting the effectiveness of the family as a nurturing and supportive group for its members, especially by intervening during family crises. I illustrated this thesis by showing how the family physician could mobilize the husband and the rest of the family in supporting the pregnant woman; and I emphasized that the doctor's efforts should not be restricted to emotional support but should have a strong cognitive component through the medium of anticipatory guidance and his advice on crisis management. I also used the crisis of bereavement as an example of the kind of opportunity presented by the daily work of physicians in preventing emotional disorder. Finally, as in the lecture about nurses, I made the point that it is necessary to provide help for the helpers; but because of the special cultural characteristics of physicians, I emphasized that the doctor himself must be active in recruiting a suitable mental health consultant for himself and in training him to offer the right kind of interprofessional support.

Chapter VII, which is a recent lecture, provides a change of pace, but is very much related to our major topic. It is an analysis of the social system and culture of schools as institutions exerting a potent effect on the psychological development of students, and it examines the implications of the values and practices of educators as role models. Here I broadened my conceptual approach from one where the caregiver operates as an individual, even when he seeks to achieve a widespread effect in a population through acting as a consultant to policy makers or to a network of caregivers, to one where the caregiver is a member of a collectivity which in toto exerts a potent influence on the entire population of an institution. This approach is in line with some of my thoughts in Chapter

I about the development of an ideology and reference group throughout the Episcopal Church that provides a supportive matrix for all its clergy.

In Chapter VIII my lecture, although delivered eight years ago, provided a contemporary-sounding, systematic pulling-together of most of the conceptual strands already discussed into a model for a comprehensive community program for preventing mental disorders. I discussed the use of the public health model of primary, secondary, and tertiary prevention in relation to mental health. I also explicated both the model of the community providing long-term supplies to a population, in order to satisfy the basic psychological needs of individuals on a wide-spread scale, and the short-term model of crisis and crisis-intervention. The chapter emphasized the value of focusing particular attention on populations at special risk, such as the aged and adolescents, and of providing a supportive structure as well as improved opportunities for need-satisfaction.

In this Chapter I showed how the above conceptual models could be used systematically in planning a comprehensive preventive program geared to pressing on all available leverage points, and using not only mental health specialists and the various networks of community caregiving professionals, but also the nonprofessional caregivers. This discussion provides the first important mention of the role of mutual-help groups in filling the gaps between the domains of professional agencies or occasioned by the shortage of professionals in some communities. The lecture also deals with informal caregivers as an important special category of helpers to people in crisis, and it advocates trying to improve their performance by educating them through the mass media.

Chapter IX is based on a lecture I delivered in 1972. Once again it focused on the role of nurses, but this time

I used the opportunity of talking to an audience of this profession to spell out a model of an organized program for the delivery of comprehensive services to cater to the entire range of needs people commonly feel. I include this lecture about changing health services within a framework of a human services philosophy in this book because I would like the concept of support systems to be seen in perspective as only part, albeit an important part, of our large field.

Finally, Chapter X presents a short lecture that summarizes my whole approach to the use of conceptual models. It represents my "model of models," and its crucial message is that since we are grappling with a highly complex multifactorial field, no single model can be expected to do more than focus our attention and pattern our expectations about one aspect of this field. If we wish to operate in a sophisticated manner in a variety of situations, we therefore need to develop and refine a series of models that we utilize in a differentiated way to complement each other.

I use conceptual models in my research and practice much as a professional photographer uses his collection of cameras and optical systems. For each situation and lighting pattern he uses a particular camera system which he has learned from experience will give him an excellent picture. In comparison with an amateur who has a limited supply of instruments or who does not know exactly how to use those he has, the professional will produce pictures of a consistent high quality, irrespective of the complexity of the field of forces with which he is confronted.

In a similar way I make use of my different models, each of which brings certain issues and situations into clear focus and obscures others. I value both the clarity of the foreground and the obscurity of the background. My total collection of models should provide me with guidance in collecting and ordering information about all the situations I normally confront. Unfortunately this is more an ideal than an actuality, and so I am continually on the lookout for additional models to add to my collection —especially for those which cut across the focal planes of my existing ones. Returning to my photography analogy, the latter are from this point of view like new lens systems, filter combinations, or improved films that can be used in the old cameras.

I believe that support systems has the makings of such a special model. It should certainly not replace the others, but it should complement and enrich them. I hope that readers of this book, particularly those who re-read Chapter I after they have read the other chapters, will be able to confirm this.

Finally, I hope my model of models explains why I have included in this book lectures which appear to overlap. They actually do overlap to some extent, and I apologize to those readers who are bored by this. But I am continually striving to examine my subject from different complementary points of view and to illuminate different facets. I hope that readers who realize the significance of this will excuse the imperfections of my method and will experience the multifactorial, multidimensional perception that I have tried to evoke.

Reference

Caplan, G. *The theory and practice of mental health consultation.* New York: Basic Books, 1970.

1

Support Systems*

The epidemiologist John C. Cassel (1973) has recently reviewed a large body of human and animal research linking increased population density, rapid social change, and social disorganization with enhanced susceptibility to disease. He has demonstrated that these researches support the hypothesis that

> *The circumstances in which increased susceptibility to disease would occur would be those in which, for a variety of reasons, individuals are not receiving any evidence (feedback) that their actions are leading to desirable and/or anticipated consequences.

The essential pathogenic element appears to be that relevant messages about expectations and evaluations of an individual's behavior are not being consistently communicated, or else that the individual is unfamiliar with expectations and the evaluative cues of those around him—including the signals that enable him to anticipate the friendliness or hostility of others. He is consequently never able to feel safe and valued, and his autonomic

*Keynote address to Conference of Department of Psychiatry, Rutgers Medical School, and New Jersey Mental Health Association on June 8, 1972, at Newark, New Jersey.

nervous system and hormonal mechanisms are continually in a state of emergency arousal, so that the resulting physiological depletion and fatigue increase his susceptibility to a wide range of physical and mental disorders.

Factors in Western urban society which increase this danger are the size, congestion, and complex organization of urban populations, and the necessity for people to travel great distances in order to maintain their daily life, all of which bring them into frequent contact with strangers; absence of generally accepted cultural norms because of heterogeneity of populations and cultural and racial conflict; population movement related to rapid socioeconomic change and greater ease of transportation; and the growth of large, complicated, and impersonal institutions that intimately affect the lives of people who do not understand how they operate.

Sir Geoffrey Vickers (1971), that most perceptive philosopher of modern society, recently formulated the crucial problem of our times as follows:

> Energy, mankind's most ancient limitation, is for the moment superabundant, and so are the means for sending messages. But the means for interpreting messages are in total confusion; and in consequence all the relations on which human life depends, at every level from the planetary to the personal, in every aspect from the economic to the ethical, are in danger of dissolution, because the regulative standards on which they depend have become confused or polarized in conflict.
>
> So the major threat at every level is the lack of what I have called an appreciative system sufficiently widely shared to mediate communication, sufficiently apt to guide action and sufficiently acceptable to make personal experience bearable. The major need

of collective existence at the moment is to generate such a system.

Cassel (1973) has shown that the risk to health posed by inconsistent or incomprehensible feedback is not shared equally by all members of a population. For instance, in animal research,

> Systematic and regular differences have been observed with the more dominant animals showing the least effects and the subordinate ones having the most extreme responses. These differences are manifest both in the magnitude of the endocrine changes as well as in increased morbidity and mortality rates.

Cassel then goes on to examine a variety of protective factors that also serve to determine which members of a population remain healthy, "those devices which 'buffer' or 'cushion' the individual from the physiological or psychological consequences of social disorganization." He suggests that these are of two main types: biological, which are related to the fundamental capacity of all living organisms to adjust physiologically and psychologically, with the passage of time, to a wide variety of environmental circumstances, so that those individuals who in the past have learned to adapt are more likely to master a current hazard; and protective social processes. Among the latter, the most significant are "the nature and strength of available group supports."

Cassell does not go into detail, but a consideration of his central thesis leads us to the conclusion that the harmful effect of absent or confusing feedback in a general population may be reduced in the case of those individuals who are effectively embedded in their own smaller social networks which provide them with consistent communications of what is expected of them, supports and assistance with tasks, evaluations of their performance, and appropriate rewards. If these are not provided by society as a whole, they can be obtained from a social subgroup. This idea is in line with the results of some of my studies (1964), of individual responses during crisis which repeatedly demonstrate that the outcome is influenced not only by the nature and vicissitudes of the stress and by the current ego strength of the individual, but, most important, by the quality of the emotional support and task-oriented assistance provided by the social network within which that individual grapples with the crisis event.

In this chapter I do not intend to focus on the central problem posed by Vickers of improving the quality of feedback to an entire population (for instance, by developing counter-cultures or new forms of institutions that cater adequately to the personal needs of all), but with the secondary issue of the discrete social supportive mechanisms that may enable certain individuals to maintain themselves in relative health and comfort in our noxious environment. By this focus I do not wish to give the impression that I favor the continuation of the harmful aspects of our current society and its institutions. I am simply choosing to deal with one of the ways of counteracting them; and, as will shortly become apparent, a way that offers the hope of widespread results.

The Nature of Support Systems

From the point of view of our present thesis, I am focusing attention on continuing social aggregates that provide individuals with opportunities for feedback about themselves and for validations of their expectations about others, which may offset deficiencies in these communications within the larger community context. But as we proceed to study such social aggregates, as Weiss (1969) did, we must take into account that most of them are initiated and maintained for other reasons, too. People have a variety of specific needs that demand satisfaction through enduring interpersonal relationships, such as for love and affection, for intimacy that provides the freedom to express feelings easily and unself-consciously, for validation of personal identity and worth, for satisfaction of nurturance and dependency, for help with tasks, and for support in handling emotion and controlling impulses. Most people develop and maintain a sense of well-being by involving themselves in a range of relationships in their lives that in toto satisfy these specific needs, such as: marriage, parenthood, other forms of loving and intimate ties, friendships, relationships with colleagues at work, membership in religious congregations and in social, cultural, political, and recreational associations, and acquaintanceships with neighbors, shopkeepers, and providers of services; intermittent relationships of help-seeking from professional caregivers such as doctors, nurses, lawyers and social workers; and continuing dependence for education and guidance on teachers, clergymen, intellectuals, and community leaders, and men of authority and influence. I am focusing special attention on certain aspects of some of these relationships, because of their significance for our present topic without, of course, implying that I am presenting an all-inclusive analysis of the meaning and significance of social ties and groupings.

The characteristic attribute of those social aggregates that act as a buffer against disease is that in such relationships, the person is dealt with as a unique individual. The other people are interested in him in a personalized way. They speak his language. They tell him what is expected of him and guide him in what to do. They watch what he does and they judge his performance. They let him know how well he has done. They reward him for success and punish or support and comfort him if he fails. Above all, they are sensitive to his personal needs, which they deem worthy of respect and satisfaction.

Such support may be of a continuing nature mediated by an enduring set of relationships with one or more significant others or groups that help the individual deal with the general issues of life or that provide special assistance in dealing with particular long-term burdens or privations. The support may also be intermittent and short-term and may be utilized from time to time by the individual in the event of an acute need or crisis. Both enduring and short-term supports are likely to consist of three elements: the significant others help the individual mobilize his psychological resources and master his emotional burdens; they share his tasks; and they provide him with extra supplies of money, materials, tools, skills, and cognitive guidance to improve his handling of his situation.

From the point of view of buffering the individual against the burden of defective feedback in the general community, support systems may operate in two ways. They may collect and store information about cues in the outside world and offer guidance and direction to the individual so that they help him to find safe paths to travel and assist him to interpret, in a balanced reality-based way, feedback cues that would otherwise be incomprehensible to him. And they may act as a refuge or sanctuary to which the individual may return for rest and recuperation in between his sorties into the stressful environment —a kind of island of stability and comfort in the turbulent sea of daily life. An individual who is lucky enough to have several supportive groups strategically situated in the community, at home, at work, in church, and in a series of recreational sites, may move from one to the other throughout the day, and be almost entirely buffered against the stressful world.

The idea that a person receives support or is in need of support usually carries the connotation that he is weak. From this point of view our term is unfortunate, because what we have in mind is not the propping up of someone who is in danger of falling down but rather the augmenting of a person's strengths to facilitate his mastery of his environment. I use the term "system" to emphasize that we mean more than an occasional or fortuitous relationship or aspect of a social association. Support *system* implies an enduring pattern of continuous or intermittent ties that play a significant part in maintaining the psychological and physical integrity of the individual over time. The various elements of the support system may be spontaneous, that is, not organized in a planned way by someone who is interested in promoting the health of the individual or the population, but emerging from the needs of the individual and the natural biosocial responses of the people in his community or from the values and traditions of his culture and society. In an unorganized or disorganized society such spontaneous support systems may be inadequate, especially for marginal people. And it is particularly in such situations and for such people that community-based feedback is likely to be insufficient and the need for individual-oriented support systems greatest. So in these cases the risk of illness will be highest unless someone takes special steps to organize a planned support system to fill the gap.

The people who are most likely to be interested in doing this are either people who have suffered and wish to help others avoid such difficulties or else the community caregiving professionals who are searching for ways of raising the level of health in the population. It must already be clear that this is a most promising approach for us. But we must be careful how we proceed, because support systems are not a professional modality and they differ in essential aspects of their operation from the helping process that we are used to seeing when a caregiving professional deals individually or in a group with lay clients. We must therefore study carefully what happens in spontaneously-arising support systems and in those systems which are organized by nonprofessionals, or those we organize using care to avoid imposing our professional stamp. By such study we may learn how to stimulate and foster supports in the population without distorting and inhibiting their development by forcing them into our professional patterns.

Spontaneous or Natural Support Systems

The best known and most ubiquitous support system in all societies is the marital and family group. Most cultures develop definite rules that legislate the reciprocal obligations that bind kinsfolk together, irrespective of their individual feelings about each other; and the more hazardous the ecological situation, the more stringent these obligations become, so people can always rely on being controlled, helped, and guided by their kin whenever they get into difficulties. Likewise they are obliged to offer similar assistance to other family members whenever the latter are in need, despite the possible personal inconvenience involved.

In our own urban society the effective whittling down of the kinship obligations of the marital couple and the nuclear family is supposed to be compensated for by the development of community caregiving agencies, manned by professionals who are especially skilled in support, and also by the mastery of the environment by urban technology so that individuals are not confronted by many life problems they must deal with on their own. Clearly, both these implicit assumptions of modern urban society are of questionable validity, and the nuclear family is usually under strain in coping with the consequent frequent demands for support by its members.

It is of interest that a number of studies, such as those by Young and Willmott (1957), of working-class families in big cities have recently shown that extended kinship networks held together by powerful bonds of mutual obligation are still in existence among the deprived members of the population who are beset by most problems and to whom the supports of the professional caregiving network are least accessible.

The essential elements in a marital or family group, from the point of view of its acting as a support system, are attitudes of sensitivity and respect for the needs of all its members and an effective communication system. It is significant that in most cases where individuals have not been protected from illness, and have therefore become accessible to study in our clinics and hospitals, their families have shortcomings in both these aspects. Disorders in marital and parent-child relationships whereby an individual is not perceived as a person in his own right whose idiosyncratic needs are worthy of assessment and satisfaction but serves as a displacement object or scapegoat for vicariously satisfying the needs of other family members are commonplace in our clinical practice. Likewise, disorders of family communication such as double binds and mystification are a usual finding in our clinical cases. We often think of these distortions of relationship and communication as directly pathogenic, but our present thesis raises the possibility of conceptualizing them also as defects in the family support system that have failed to protect the individuals from the effects of inadequate feedback in the outside world.

A fascinating reflection on the significance of the family pattern as a basic support system is provided by the frequent finding that individuals who, for a variety of reasons, do not have a family of their own often are "adopted" by a family to which they are not linked by birth or marriage. This applies not only to children who are formally adopted or fostered, but also to adults. Another version of the same theme has been described by Joan Shapiro (1971) in her sensitive study of people living as single-room occupants in low-cost rooming houses in New York City. She found that in many of these dilapidated hotels the poverty-stricken inmates spontaneously cluster together in enduring pseudofamily groups, each under the leadership of a dominant woman who acts as a kind of mother who nurtures, guides, and controls those who feel bound to her. Within such a pseudofamily group a network of reciprocal kin-like obligations develops which supports and protects these erstwhile isolated derelicts against the privations of their marginal existence. The family-like groupings among adolescent hippies and dropouts, which sometimes take on a more organized pattern as in the notorious Manson Family, are a similar manifestation, attesting to the attractiveness of the family pattern to people who cluster together spontaneously for mutual support. It is worthy of note that the reason most frequently expressed verbally by such people for joining and maintaining their membership in such an aggregate is that in this group they feel that others treat them as unique individuals, try to satisfy their idiosyncratic needs, and support them lovingly in "doing their thing."

In modern English, when we wish to refer somewhat poetically to a person's relatives we sometimes use the term "kith and kin." But in Middle English and Anglo-Saxon this term differentiated two sets of people. *Kin* denoted those bound by birth or marriage, namely family members, whereas *kith* denoted friends, acquaintances, and neighbors, giving recognition to the special part played by such people in an individual's life. In its original usage *kith* represents a support system which is important for many people. This is especially so, in our society, among members of ethnic subgroups, first or second generation immigrants from rural and semi-rural settlements in Europe.

Kith bonds and supports may be weaker in this country, especially in large cities, than in rural and semi-rural Europe, but I feel that relatively superficial links with neighbors often do add up to a not insignificant system of supports. Many of us in large cities derive a special sense of community and validation of self from recognizing and being recognized by the people on our block, the man from whom we buy the newspaper, the owner of the dry-cleaning store to which we take our clothes, the corner grocer, and the drugstore owner.

Kin and kith supports mainly provide continuing guidance and direction as well as self-validation. Intermittently, they are called into operation to sustain their members in acute crisis situations or in dealing with chronic deprivation. But in confronting such out-of-the-ordinary challenges, kin and kith supports are often augmented by the special services of a network of helping people in the community whom we have named "informal caregivers." I became interested in these people when I was investigating the nature of individual responses to crisis, and found that many individuals in crisis turn to such people for help and guidance and that the outcome of the crisis is much influenced by the quality of their intervention. Robert Liberman (1965) made a similar finding when he investigated what appeared to determine whether a mentally ill person entered a mental hospital via a medical referral or via the police. He discovered that of "52 individuals who sought help 63% were influenced by another person in their choice of a particular resource." He found that the people he named "influentials" were older, less likely to be Protestant, more often of a higher socioeconomic class, higher in gregariousness, more stable residentially, and more likely to have had prior experience with mentally ill family members than those who sought their guidance.

We still await an in-depth study of such informal caregivers—it is long overdue. However, the following are my impressions of them. They are of two types, "generalists" and "specialists." The "generalists" are likely to be people who are widely recognized in their neighborhood to have wisdom in matters of human relations or to be knowledgable about the community caregiving system. As Liberman pointed out, they are gregarious; that is, they make contacts easily and like to involve themselves with other people. Often, they have a social or economic role that brings them into repetitive contact with many others; for instance, they may serve in a drug store or a grocery store, or they may be hairdressers, bar tenders, policemen, or newspaper vendors. Often they have had emotional problems themselves or have had to deal with such difficulties in their own families, and this has stimulated their interest and understanding. Some of them may appear to us to be currently disturbed and to be trying to master their own problems vicariously by intervening in the lives of others, but if they consistently give ineffectual advice they soon get a bad name in their locality and people stop paying attention to them. Whatever their motivation, these informal caregivers must demonstrate good results in order to earn and maintain the local reputation that will attract neighbors to solicit their help.

The "specialist" counsellors are rather different. They are usually people who are known to have suffered some misfortune or to have undergone a particular trying experience and to have worked out ways of achieving a successful adjustment and adaptation. Their personality gifts and interest in helping others may be of less significance than the quality of their adaptation and their demonstration of mastery over their own life difficulties, at least as this is perceived by the people around them. They are sought out by others who find themselves in the same kinds of situations and they are asked for their advice as people who have personal experience of this problem. Eventually, some of these people who have successfully handled their own predicament, and have subsequently been asked to help others with similar difficulties, discover that they enjoy this kind of service, and both they and the people who turn to them for help find that they have some interpersonal talent. They may then develop a local reputation as helpful persons, and many fellow sufferers may turn to them and may be given guidance and support.

The variety of such specialized, local, informal helpers is large; almost anyone with an illness or disability, or who is exposed to a personal or family predicament or challenge, has a tendency to seek guidance from somebody else who has travelled a similar experiential route and who can tell what to expect as well as what options have proved to be the best for grappling with the burdens and challenges. Our Harvard group (1960) has been informally studying this phenomenon for several years. When, for example, we were conducting our research on adjustment of parents to the birth of a premature baby, we were impressed by the number who actively sought advice from other parents who had earlier been through the same experience. We found that there was a positive correlation between making a special effort to look for such information from other parents and a healthy adaptation to the crisis. It appeared that information about what to expect and how to treat the baby was obtained in a more understandable and usable form from other parents than from the professionals, despite the latter's more standardized expertise and wider experience. We found similar patterns of seeking guidance from people with prior personal experience among the parents of babies with congenital defects and with mental retardation. But the best example of this phenomenon was the case of widows. My colleague, Phyllis Silverman (1969), conducted a survey of recently widowed women in order to discover whom they had found to be most helpful to them at different phases of their bereavement. She reported:

> Most caregivers shy away from the bereaved. Widows I have talked with felt that neither friends, family, physicians, nor clergymen, for that matter, were very helpful. All wanted them to recover as quickly as possible. On the other hand, they found that other widows could be extremely helpful; they were least likely to tell them to 'keep a stiff upper lip' at a time when the widows felt their lives were ended and any hope for the future gone. Other widows realized that grief was temporary and had to run its course before it was possible to feel better again.

So other widows would encourage them to weep and

would weep along with them, utilizing this as an opportunity to continue, although at a much lower intensity, their unending process of mourning for their own dead spouses. The new widows felt that the veteran widows really understood their situation as no nonwidowed person could, and that what they said was authentic because it was based on personal experience. They also saw that the other woman had survived and that, even though she continued to be faithful to her husband's memory and intermittently to mourn him, this no longer incapacitated her.

The outstanding characteristic of these informal caregivers, both generalists and specialists, is that they are nonprofessionals. They are amateurs in the fullest sense of the word. Webster defines an amateur as "a person who does something for the pleasure of it rather than for money; nonprofessional; hence, a person who does something more or less unskillfully." While it is true that compared with professionals whose performance is supposed to be standardized at a high level of skill by appropriate recruitment, training, and supervision, these amateur caregivers are quite varied, many of them are just as effective in their supportive achievements as professionals and some of them get better results because of their amateur status. For instance, the informal caregivers usually do not maintain a professional style of distance and objectivity in dealing with the people they help. Instead, the caregivers involve themselves personally with the others. They do not utilize standardized techniques, but extemporaneous expressions of their own personality. They do not empathize but they identify. All this adds up to a direct person-to-person influence which has an authenticity and spontaneity rare among professionals, except the best trained and most talented.

Another characteristic of informal caregivers is that there is a mutual and reciprocal quality in their interac-

tions with the people they help. The giver and the
receiver of support are equally, though differently,
benefited by the contact. This is especially obvious in the
case of a veteran giving counsel to a recent sufferer, when
the former plays an active role in a situation that revives
in him the memory of an experience in which previously
he himself was the relatively passive sufferer, so that he
may now exercize mastery in place of his former victimiza-
tion. This is made all the more vivid because he vicariously re-experiences the old pains and discomforts as he
identifies with the current sufferer. This identification is
overtly or covertly recognized by the sufferer, and it is
because of this recognition that he feels so well understood. This is one reason that many people prefer to get
help from a person whose expertise comes from having
personally experienced the predicament rather than from
a professional who may only have scientific knowledge of
it. They feel it is more authentic. They also feel in such
contacts that neither party is standardized, so they do not
need to feel that they are "cases," and therefore, to some
extent, "put down." While the interaction of professional
and client is hierarchical, that of the amateur supporter
and the person he is helping is coordinate. This is
emphasized by the fact that it is usually entirely voluntary
on both sides; the absence of financial payment makes it
seem a more sincere and personalized service which is
energized by true lovingkindness.

Organized Supports Not Directed by Caregiving Professionals

The second main category of supports are those that are
organized through formal groups and associations which
are established and maintained by people similar to the

informal caregivers we have just described. These organizations sometimes use caregiving professionals as resource people, and if they are big enough they may use professional administrators or other paid professional staff, but the main direction remains in the hands of the amateurs. There are two types of such organizations, the voluntary service groups and the mutual help groups.

All through history, people interested in their fellow men have banded themselves together to offer service to those in need, either for explicitly religious reasons or simply because of a personal need to serve and nurture others, the satisfaction of which lends extra meaning and fulfillment to life. A good contemporary example of such a volunteer service organization is the one initiated in 1964 in London by a group of young people under the leadership of a 27-year-old barrister, Anthony Steen. Within four years he and a group of like-minded young people, all in their twenties, built up an organization of over 10,000 volunteers between the ages of 14 and 30, who devoted themselves to serving the lonely and elderly people of London. They called their organization Task Force, and they captured the imagination of young people of all classes throughout the city. Their members conducted a house-to-house search for lonely old people and put these in touch with volunteers who were prepared to give companionship and immediate help, such as redecorating rooms, window cleaning, shopping, repairing radio and television sets, pushing wheelchairs, playing cards, hairdressing, shaving, sewing and mending, taking them to the movies or for car outings, and so on. Most important, many of the young volunteers built ongoing relationships with the elderly as proxy grandchildren, and they also brought many of the old people together into small peer groups.

The volunteers organized and staffed their own offices

in seven of the London boroughs and linked up with the municipal health and welfare services. They actively recruited other volunteers from among senior school children, university students, and in industry, as well as from churches and recreational organizations. Their success was recognized by the British Government, and in 1968 a country-wide Voluntary Community Service by Young People was established along similar lines, with the support of several Government ministries. A joint circular (1968) announcing the formation of the organization sponsored by a newly-created voluntary foundation stated in its introduction:

> The Government has been particularly impressed by the widespread enthusiasm of young people to render service to the community. They are concerned that this fund of energy and goodwill should be used to the full, so as to support the work already being done and increase the opportunities for voluntary service.

Our own Peace Corps, Vista, and local youth service organizations (such as Harvard's Philips Brooks House), and many other associations of student volunteers who serve in mental hospitals, nursing homes, settlement houses, and in outreach services to the underprivileged, are too well known to need more than brief mention. Perhaps less familiar to a mental health audience, but undeservedly so, is the volunteer service effort of people at the other end of the age scale—the American Association of Retired Persons, which currently has a membership of 3-1/2 million and which, in addition to its mutual-help activities, harnesses the tremendous energy of its countrywide membership in a wide range of local and regional service projects. It would be hard to find another organization that so aptly demonstrates the mutuality of

the benefit to helper and helped in activities providing
the opportunity for retired people to continue to fulfill
themselves in useful service to individuals, organizations,
and the general community. Clearly, in addition to the
personal significance of this service for each individual
member of this and similar organizations, and in addition
to their contribution to the community's supportive network, the association itself provides a most potent supportive matrix for its own members through their social and
organizational contacts in furthering their common cause.

The second type of supportive organizations are the
mutual help associations, some of which have a long history. The Freemasons, for instance, started in the Middle
Ages after the Black Death had devastated Europe and
destroyed much of society's supportive structure. The
organization had previously been a craft guild of stonema-
sons, but as a response to the perils and privations of the
times it reorganized to build a social matrix for its members to support themselves in withstanding the confusions
of their environment—a classic example of Cassel's thesis.

Similar organizations have emerged to support population subgroups whenever there has been rapid cultural
change or social disorganization. For instance, in countries
experiencing massive immigration, the newcomers often
band together in "landsmanschaften" or ethnic organizations, and in "fraternal" associations like Elks, Lions, or
Workingmen's Clubs. The veterans' organizations that
grow up after wars are another example. In addition to
providing a range of acceptable social activities in familiar
surroundings, most of these organizations establish group
insurance against sickness and death, as well as traditions
of helping each other in times of personal need both by
financial loans and by mutual counseling, in addition to
visiting the sick and the bereaved.

Supplementing such "generalist" organizations, we also

find mutual-help associations which are the collective analogues of the individual, specialized caregivers: organizations of people who have all suffered a particular disability or undergone a challenging experience, and which provide a structure for mutual support in withstanding deprivations, or for oldtimers to help the recent additions to their ranks. The best known example in our own days is Alcoholics Anonymous. This organization not only provides individual and group counselling by recovered alcoholics to those who are struggling to kick the habit, but actively recruits members through a kind of missionary work among alcoholics. It also offers massive social supports to its members through convivial meetings which may be attended almost every evening and at weekends and which resemble alcoholic parties, but are held without alcohol.

Alcoholics Anonymous, like many specialized mutual-help groups that help to combat addictions or actively seek to overcome deprivations, offers not only the current emotional support of social contacts but also a body of traditions and values and a system of concepts which add up to a specific life style and ideology which, in many ways, resembles a religion in providing internal psychological and spiritual supports to its members, buttressed by social rituals and ceremonials.

Alcoholics Anonymous was formed, in part, as a reaction against the ineffectiveness of professional treatment of alcoholics, and became what today we would call a counter-culture. The current increase in drug abuse and the widespread disenchantment with formal professional treatment programs has stimulated the emergence of a host of self-help groups organized by ex-addicts. Matthew Dumont (1973) has written a thoughtful study of this phenomenon.

To me, one of his most interesting findings was that the atmosphere in many of these self-help groups is explicitly authoritarian. Members are expected to adhere to a strict code of conduct, centering of course on drug abstinence. They are kept under careful surveillance and they are severely judged for backsliding, which is punished by public condemnation and shaming. On the other hand, if members keep the rules and demonstrate commitment to the social norms and traditions of the group, they are progressively elevated in status until they are admitted to the top leadership stratum, and in their turn may command the respect and obedience of those lower in the hierarchy. Dumont uses the term "paramilitary" in describing the controls and sanctions of the ex-addict organizations. To me, they also resemble religious orders in their social structure and controls. All of these institutions have in common a well-defined mission to train members and support them in a disciplined new style of life; they combine an authoritarian hierarchy with an open-ended upward-mobility system that balances punitive sanctions for nonconformity with the very tangible rewards of unlimited promotion for merit. They differ fundamentally from professional care systems in that the latter maintain a rigid boundary between the lay clients and the professional staff, and no amount of egalitarianism ever completely obscures the essentially negative judgement of the client involved.

Organizations that help their members break a noxious habit—alcoholism, drug abuse, smoking, or overeating —offer not only individual and group counselling in dealing with the problems involved and particularly anticipatory guidance from oldtimers in preparing for expectable difficulties, but they also extend individual ego strength by group sharing of the miseries and discomforts of withdrawal symptoms. In addition, they provide a community in which friendships can develop to provide a new meaning to life; also, social and recreational activities can take place that offer a distraction from the unsatisfied cravings.

Another group of organizations places its main emphasis on the provision of a new community in which members may immerse themselves. These are the organizations catering to those who have suffered a major loss or a relatively unalterable disability or deprivation, like Parents Without Partners, Widows Associations, Parents of Mentally Retarded or Psychotic Children, Mastectomy and Ileostomy Associations, Amputees, Disabled War Veterans, and so on. Most of these self-help groups have two-phase programs. The oldtimers help the new members to master the trauma of the acute crisis of the bereavement, the loss of bodily integrity, or the disappointment of parental hopes, by means of individual and group counselling and by emotional support in expressing and mastering the shock and pain, as well as by guidance in accepting and coming to terms with the catastrophe. But the characteristic feature of these organizations is their second-phase provision of long-term social contacts and joint activities which serve as a kind of psychosocial replacement for what has been lost. This never really works—no amount of friendliness in meetings of Parents Without Partners can replace the intimacy of a marital relationship, nor can collaborating with other parents in bettering the lot of the mentally retarded make up for the life-long feeling of emptiness caused by having a child who will never develop to continue the chain of one's life. But at least the association with others in the same situation combats the social isolation that would otherwise be the lot of those who feel themselves, and are perceived by others, to be deviant in ordinary society.

A characteristic feature of many of the organizations of

the deprived is that they develop cohesion and some sense of mastery over cruel fate by campaigning politically for improvement of the community's handling of the needs of people like themselves. The outstanding example of this has been the activism of associations of parents of the retarded, which has been very successful in forcing authorities to provide radical improvements in the care of their children. In the process they have emerged from their previous shame-burdened obscurity and ineffectuality into players of powerful roles on the community stage, and this has given them self-respect and a deeply meaningful experience of channeling their frustrated nurturance into a useful cause.

I will mention only one of the other characteristics of many of these mutual-help groups of "people in the same boat." They not only offer each other emotional and social supports and opportunities, but they usually provide detailed information and specific guidance in increasing their members' understanding of the issues involved in their predicament and of practical ways of dealing with the expectable day-to-day and long-term problems. This cognitive input is usually provided in a highly structured way through the medium of discussion groups moderated by the oldtimers who share the benefits of their experience with the new members. A good example of this is found in the activities of La Leche League, a mutual-help organization of nursing mothers which was started by a few women in Chicago in the late 1950's and now has over a thousand groups of members in this country, as well as branches overseas.

The following account is by Mrs. Hope Murrow, a Fellow of the Harvard Laboratory of Community Psychiatry, who is studying this organization:

The usual La Leche League group consists of 10-30

mothers from a geographic area. Members learn of
the organization through doctors, nurses, friends, and
newspaper announcements. There is a series of four
highly structured meetings which is repeated several
times during the year. The topics of these meetings
are (1) advantages of nursing; (2) overcoming difficulties in nursing; (3) baby arrives and joins the family (including a discussion of labor and birth); (4) nutrition and weaning (including understanding of tod-
dler and sibling rivalry). The atmosphere of the meetings I have attended is almost of a religious nature,
with the goal of inspiring and re-dedicating women
in their commitment to motherhood. Attending the
meeting are pregnant women, new mothers with
infants, and those with several older children. After
the formal part of the meeting, there is much informal conversation about specific problems and solutions. Each group maintains a full library of articles
and books on childbirth, nursing, and childrearing.
Each member receives a regular newsletter. Group
leaders are available for telephone consultation at any
time, and in turn may receive advice from other
knowledgable people within the system. Referrals are
made, on occasion, to doctors and other professionals.
Women are encouraged to consult with others in
their own situation.

New group leaders are chosen carefully, after their
functioning within the group and relationships with
their own children are observed over a period of
time. They then enter into a period of training which
involves reading, and discussions with experienced
leaders, as well as workshops. The system is very well
organized, and maintains central control with regional
and state coordination, and a central office in
Chicago.

Religious Denominations as Organized Support Systems

Unfortunately, shortage of space permits only the briefest mention of a most important topic. This topic deserves a whole chapter to itself, since religious denominations are the most widely available organized support systems in the community and probably cater on a regular basis to more people than all the others.

Setting aside the primary theological aspects of religions for the purpose of this discussion, what impresses me most about them are the following support system charac-teristics: Most denominations are organized in congregations of neighbors. They hold regular meetings and provide a range of opportunities for their members to become friends and to identify with each other. This process is fostered by their joint allegiance to a shared theology and to a common value system and body of traditions. Members are usually enjoined to help each other, especially in times of acute need; religious ceremonials as well as service programs are provided to accomplish this, especially at predictable crisis times such as birth, marriage, illness, and death. These organized social supports are significantly buttressed by the internal supports of a meaningful value system and set of guidelines for living, so that the religious person does not feel that he is dependent only on his individual wisdom in grappling with life's problems. He can rely on the wisdom of the ages enshrined in his religion. He can also rely on the positive and negative sanctions of a present and cohesive reference group to help him control and direct his impulses and chart his course in life.

Most religions organize regular and frequent opportunities for reinforcement of these supports, both through individual daily prayer that links the person with all the others who share his faith and through daily or weekly religious services that utilize rituals and ceremonies which are most powerful evokers of group identification and cohesion. The readings from the holy books as well as the sermons on such occasions strengthen the cognitive bonds among the members by adding to their shared values and world views, and they also help each person to articulate his current experience with the wisdom and traditions of his denomination. They reinforce a faith in God that gives meaning to life and hope for a better future.

Clearly, a religious person who is an active member of a local congregation is powerfully buffered against defects in feedback in the general population, and this is especially so during crisis periods. Moreover, if he belongs to a large denomination he is likely to find a welcoming congregation with familiar rituals and traditions in any new and strange place to which he may go. This will protect him until he learns the local feedback cues and will support his adjustment even if the general social structure is disorganized.

Contributions of Community Mental Health Professionals

What I have discussed so far leads me to conclude that professionals interested in preventing mental disorder and promoting mental health on a widespread scale in a population should devote significant effort to fostering the development of support systems of all kinds in the communities they serve. Until recently, we paid little attention to this topic as a central issue, although many of us have done some of this kind of work in an unplanned way. I believe that over the next decade the field will become

a major focus of systematic research. Meanwhile, the following comments are based on some initial explorations
of the past few years.

Community mental health specialists may make their
contributions in four main ways: First, by initiating or
helping to organize new support systems inside community institutions; second, by organizing new support systems in the outside community; third, by offering consultation and education to the organizers and other key members of existing organized support systems; and, fourth,
by offering consultation to members of unorganized supportive networks in the community.

Organizing a New Support System Inside an Institution

An excellent example of such a system is a project our
Harvard Laboratory of Community Psychiatry has been
conducting over the past five years in the Episcopal
Church. A full account of it is contained in a book that
has just been completed by Ruth Caplan (1972), the title
of which epitomizes the goal of our efforts in this entire
field. The book is called *Helping the Helpers to Help*. It
describes how we set up a consultation program in the
Diocese of Massachusetts consisting of two consultation
groups for parish clergy that have been meeting weekly
and discussing current work problems with individual
parishioners and their families and with the organization
of the parish. The program also includes regular consultation sessions with the Bishop and his headquarters staff
that focus on problems of administering the Diocese and
providing counsel and support to the parish clergy. During the past three years this Massachusetts project has
been extended to a country-wide program through the
medium of the Pastoral Development Committee of the
Episcopal House of Bishops. I have acted as a resource

specialist to this Committee in helping them organize a program that they have named Bishop-to-Bishop Coordinate Status Consultation. I have trained a cadre of 23 experienced bishops in consultation techniques; now every newly-consecrated bishop in the Church is offered the opportunity of choosing a consultant from this group who will help him grapple constructively with the difficulties and challenges of his first two years in office, with particular reference to organizing a supportive structure in his diocese to foster the pastoral work of his parish clergy. This bishop-to-bishop consultation program is going well; I meet regularly twice a year for two-day supervisory group meetings with the consultant bishops. Bishop David E. Richards, a senior bishop who is the Executive Secretary of the Pastoral Development Committee, undertakes the staff work to weld this program together. With my help he has made a special study of consultation techniques, and he offers advice and counsel to the consultant bishops on the day-to-day technical and organizational aspects of the program. I am available by telephone to any consultant who desires special supervisory advice.

My work with Bishop Richards has brought into focus the importance of using one or more key staff of an institution as intermediaries in organizing such a support system. Outside specialists can exert great leverage in establishing programs, but the innumerable practicalities of maintaining an ongoing operation demand an inside man with authority and influence, and with the detailed knowledge of the workings of the organization. I plan eventually to move out of the Episcopal Church program and to hand over my role entirely to Bishop Richards, whom I am, in a way, coaching to serve as my replacement. Hopefully this will ensure that the program will become a permanent feature in the structure of the Church.

When we started this work we conceptualized it simply as offering mental health consultation to a group of significant caregiving professionals. But as we proceeded, we began to realize that we were involved in a much more important undertaking, and we began to mold our operations accordingly. The Church, mainly through its parish clergy, touches the lives of a vast population of parishioners and their families, and is involved in all the strains of our current turbulent world. What our program is doing is helping the clergy to deal with the mental health dimension of their complicated task through stimulating the building in of a network of individual, group, and administrative supports at key levels within the structure of their church organization to augment those that are already in existence. We mental health specialists are an important element in this operation, but its essential core is the organized network of mutual influences of the bishops and their clergy.

Our experience so far indicates the following issues to have been significant:

Improvement in Mental Health Knowledge and Skills. An important contribution of our mental health specialists was to communicate to bishops and parish clergy cognitive content about mental health, patterns of crisis coping, methods of crisis intervention, ways of assessing and managing cases of mental disturbance in parishioners and their families, and ways of identifying and satisfying the psychosocial needs of individuals and groups, both clergy and parishioners. We demonstrated the importance of systematic continuing education about such topics at all levels of the organization, much of which can be accomplished just as well by educators on the staff of the Church as by outside consultants.

Provision of Authoritative Consultation. Our consultants were accepted as experts in their field, and it was a source of great support to have them available as authorities to whom the clergy and their leaders could turn for guidance in an emergency and on whom they could rely for clarifying their confusions. We hope that eventually Bishop Richards and his colleagues may organize a cadre of psychologically trained churchmen who will replace us in this expert role so that they can integrate in the same authority figures both mental health expertise and leadership in their religion.

Peer Supports. The third source of support in our program were the peer groups that we organized both for parish clergy and for experienced bishops. We hope shortly also to arrange discussions among consultee bishops, and by this means to develop a continuing peer group structure for them. The benefits from a peer group are two-fold. It provides social-emotional supports of regular friendly interaction with those in similar situations who understand one's predicaments and share one's concerns. And it offers help with current tasks provided by those who describe how they have handled similar situations and what the consequences were of different ways of dealing with them. Our experience leads us to the conclusion that these coordinate status groups do best if they are moderated by an outside leader of higher status who can help the members evaluate themselves and each other constructively, so that when they are under stress they may pull each other up rather than down.

Reference Group Supports. The fourth and most powerful element of our program has been the development of reference groups among the parish clergy and the bishops with whom we have worked. We have helped these people build up an ideology in such matters as emphasizing the importance of a calm methodical analysis of a confusing situation, avoidance of premature judgments because of frustration, and the belief that the most apparently inexplicable human behavior can be understood if we investigate enough intrasystemic and intersystemic connections among the phenomena of the case. What emerges is a shared style of methodical problem solving and of testing the reality of perceptions and expectations in emotionally arousing work situations.

Here, too, our mental health workers have initiated a process that can be perfectly well continued by the church leaders on their own, the goal being the development of a church culture that prescribes normative behavior and ways of problem solving in mental health matters with which all clergymen can identify when grappling with the human predicaments of their work.

Among other projects which operate along somewhat similar lines I have time only to mention one. Beatrix A. Hamburg, a child psychiatrist, and Barbara B. Varenhorst, a psychologist (1972), have recently initiated a most interesting program of peer counselling in the secondary schools of Palo Alto, California. They recruited 160 children from grades 7-12, using the self-selection approach of soliciting volunteers. They organized a course of ten training sessions for those volunteers, which was highly structured and made considerable demands on the capacities and commitment of the participants with the result that the less suitable weeded themselves out. The training was accomplished through lectures, seminars, role playing exercises, and supervised practicum; key educators from the school system collaborated with the mental health specialists, so that in future programs they will be able to handle this phase on their own. The practicum consisted of sending trainees to visit elementary schools in May and June to offer counselling to groups of sixth graders who were preparing for the move to junior high school, and who were told that the peer counsellor would be available to them on arrival at their junior high school in the fall.

It is too early to evaluate the achievements of this program, but its approach and style fit neatly into the conceptual model of building a support system within an institution. Hamburg and Varenhorst see their project as the initial stage of a comprehensive school mental health plan:

> The long-range objective is to develop a totally self-sustaining peer counselling program which can function effectively within a school system with a minimum necessity for involvement of outside mental health professionals.

They plan to train teachers and counsellors to carry on the program and in so doing improve their own general mental health skills. And they hope to find a school administrator who will take over the continuing organization, much as Bishop Richards is doing in our Church program.

Organizing a New Support System in the "Open Community"

In this age of "de-institutionalization" when there is a search for viable alternatives to traditional institutions for satisfying health and welfare needs, many mental health professionals are establishing free-standing support systems in the manner of the spontaneously occurring mutual help organizations. A good example is our Harvard Widow-to-Widow program.[10] This was established by Phyllis Silverman in 1967 as a result of a survey, to which I have previously referred, which revealed that most widows are not being adequately helped by existing community agencies and caregiving professionals. Accordingly, in collaboration with representatives of several of the local social agencies, she set up a pilot program in Dorchester, a racially and religiously mixed section of Boston. She recruited five widows, who were drawn from the dominant religious and racial groups in the community, to serve as aides. These women had no special educational background but were chosen because they had already demonstrated skill and local acceptability as informal caregivers, and because they seemed to have successfully mastered the problems of their own widowhood. We obtained the names and addresses of all men under 60 who had died recently in Dorchester from death certificates received from the Bureau of Vital Statistics, and we then got information on their race and religion from funeral directors. The aides were given this information and they systematically contacted and offered help to widows of the same race and religion as themselves. The majority of the new widows accepted the help through the medium of personal visits by the aide or of telephone conversations with her.

Dr. Silverman convened a meeting of the aides group once a week to talk over their experience, but she made no attempt to "train" them, nor to interfere with their nonprofessional ways of helping. Instead, she studied how they dealt with situations on the basis of their personal experience and native gifts. She found that they provided emotional support, friendship, concrete service such as help in finding a job or going with the new widow to agency offices, and information about such matters as bereavement, widowhood, care of children in the absence of a father, and how to manage the home finances.

After about a year the aides found that their case loads were growing too big to handle by one-to-one methods, particularly as they never "closed a case," but reduced their contacts in line with feelings of lessened need of the widows. The aides then began to supplement their individual contacts with a variety of group interactions. They convened meetings of special interest groups to discuss such topics as job retraining, child care, and financial problems. They also organized social and recreational groups and small friendship groups of widows with similar interests. They stimulated the development of mutual-help groups for widows in religious and other community organizations. Eventually they organized a self-help group for widows and widowers in the Greater Boston region by recruiting a core group of volunteers who established a 24-hour-a-day telephone counselling service. This has led to the development of a network of mutual-help groups throughout our area; the original widow-aides are now operating as educators and supervisors of the volunteers who function as leaders in these ventures.

Our local program has aroused considerable interest among widows throughout the country; and recent developments include Dr. Silverman and the widow-aides organizing two conferences attended by people from many states who wish to establish similar projects in their own area, and an approach by a large national organization of retired persons which is negotiating with them to develop a mutual help program for the widowed among their members.

In reviewing this program we should realize that Dr. Silverman as its professional initiator played a most important role. She pinpointed the problem and derived the overall pattern of solution. She recruited the aides. She selected and convened the policy-setting and sanctioning group of community agency representatives. She negotiated with the Bureau of Vital Statistics to obtain the death certificates and with the funeral directors to get supplementary information about the bereaved. Through our Harvard framework she legitimated the functioning of the aides vis-à-vis the community authorities—a not insignificant matter, since they had no formal qualifications as caregivers and two of them had not been educated beyond the eighth grade. She moderated and guided the weekly aides meetings. She encouraged and counselled the aides, especially in the early stages of the program when they still lacked confidence. She was continually present in the background, holding a watching brief, and immediately available to bail out anyone in difficulty. She exercised leadership in moving from Dorchester to Greater Boston and then to a country-wide program. She was the prime mover, in collaboration with me, in securing funds for the project which involved obtaining university and National Institute of Mental Health sanction and support. But she did not establish the policies of the program; that was done by the Dorchester agency representatives originally, and later by the committees of the successive widow organizations. And she did not direct the day-to-day operations of the program, or prescribe ways of handling the cases; that was accomplished by the aides themselves. Nor did she train the aides in methods and techniques derived from her professional background. Whenever the aides asked questions about scientific or community organizational and administrative matters, she answered them; but mainly she acted as an enabler to foster their own development of amateur ways of dealing with the challenges of their role, and these varied considerably from aide to aide in line with each person's idiosyncratic experiences and capacities.

Consultation to an Already Organized Support Group

This type of work involves the professional in operations as an outsider invited in to fulfill a requested role within an organized informal community support group, similar to what he does as a consultant in a formal community agency or institution. A good example is the work of Norris Hansell (1971) with the Looking Glass of Chicago. The latter is an organization of about forty volunteers with a full-time nonprofessional staff of five which offers counselling and information services to late adolescents and young adults who have left home and are in distress in the Chicago area. They serve about 500 persons a year who usually find out about them through word of mouth. Their clients are mostly alienated young persons who do not wish to contact the formal care-giving agencies of the community, young people who have run away from home toward the Chicago bright lights.

Hansell was asked to develop a training program for new volunteer staff and to help existing staff learn from their own experience. He accomplished these goals by a series of six discussions. In his own words,

> The group presents a problem. We discuss it together. I attempt to summarize the discussion and get their critique of the summary. *We work to select, from what they have said, the active ingredients in the process they describe, and to separate out what is trivial and irrelevant.*

As a result of this series of discussions, Hansell was able to help the Looking Glass group explicate the regularly-occurring aspects of their counselling and develop a set of guidelines for new members that put the ideology of the organization into words and made explicit the style of its helping operations. In Hansell's words, this was summarized as follows:

> Receive the client. Define help. Offer Help. Define a discrete task. Use cognitively-oriented counselling. Focus on decisions. Maintain a relationship

with other Looking Glass staff for corporate scrutiny of service. Link unlinked clients to persons in similar status in Chicago. Maintain an average transit time in service of six weeks or less. Techniques include anticipatory guidance; mourning counselling; diverting an individual from his topic of choice; and converting the laundry list of complaints into a specification of excellence and strategy for improvement.

In his report on this work Hansell writes,

> It is my overall impression that Looking Glass is doing a better job with the risk group with which they deal than a professional agency would likely do. In addition, they are seeing a group that does not come to professional agencies. They have evolved a method close to what I call 'decision counselling' and have aspects of what I call the 'spin-off group' method.

It is easy to understand that the communication of such opinions by a high-status professional is a source of great support to a group of amateur volunteers who do not have the benefit of professional guild standards against which to evaluate their own achievements.

Fostering Already Existing Unorganized Supportive Services

In many neighborhoods the kith supports, although not circumscribed and organized, add up to a widespread support system that is often implicitly recognized as such by the local inhabitants who know to whom to turn for help in times of need, or whom to ask for guidance about sources of help. Mental health professionals may study this naturally-occurring system and may then take steps to foster and augment it. Alice Collins (1972) has provided us with a good model of how to accomplish this in the child day care field. She and her professional colleagues in Portland, Oregon explore a neighborhood in order to identify the female informal caregivers, whom they call "natural neighbors." From among the latter they identify those who are already involved in child day-care activities and augment their number by recruiting additional caregivers. The mental health workers then develop an ongoing consultation relationship with this group and foster their specialization in day care and they extend the number of families each serves to about 50-75. Alice Collins and her colleagues have found that a single mental health worker can offer effective consultation on an individual basis to about 15 day care neighbors and so can affect the lives of about 750-1,000 families. A basic principle of their approach is to recognize and show appropriate respect for the natural skills of the nonprofessional day care neighbors. The professionals do not denigrate them by offering to "train" them. Instead, they offer them classical consultee-centered case consultations within the framework of a coordinate relationship, much as mental health consultants are accustomed to do with non-mental health professionals.

References

Caplan, G. Patterns of parental response to the crisis of premature birth: A preliminary approach to modifying mental health outcome. *Psychiatry*, 1960, 23, 365-374.

Caplan, G. *Principles of preventive psychiatry*. New York: Basic Books, 1964.

Caplan, R. *Helping the helpers to help.* New York: Sea-
bury Press, 1972.

Cassel, J. C. Psychiatric epidemiology. In G. Caplan
(Ed.), *American handbook of psychiatry.* Vol. II.
New York: Basic Books, in press 1973.

Collins, A. H. Natural delivery systems: Accessible
sources of power for mental health. Paper presented
at the 49th Annual Meeting of the American Ortho-
psychiatric Association, Detroit, April, 1972.

Dumont, M. P. Drug problems and their treatment. In
G. Caplan (Ed.), *American handbook of psychiatry.*
Vol. II. New York: Basic Books, in press 1973.

Hamburg, B. A. & Varenhorst, B. A. A community mental health project for youth: Peer counselling in the
secondary schools. *American Journal of Orthopsychiatry,* 1972, 42, 566-581.

Hansell, N. Exploration of service methods of a volunteer
counselling group. Discussions with staff of Looking
Glass of Chicago. Northwestern University Medical
School, Department of Psychiatry, unpublished man-
uscript, 1971.

Joint circular, Department of Education and Science,
Ministry of Health, Home Office, Ministry of Housing and Local Government. London: April, 1968.

Liberman, R. Personal influence in the use of mental
health resources. *Human Organization,* 1965, 24,
231-235.

Shapiro, J. H. *Communities of the alone.* New York:
Association Press, 1971.

Silverman, P. R. The widow-to-widow program. An
experiment in preventive intervention. *Mental Hygiene,* 1969, 53, 333-337.

Vickers, G. Institutional and personal roles. *Human Relations,* 1971, XXIV, 433-447.

Webster's New World dictionary of the American language. Cleveland & New York: World Publishing Co., 1964.

Weiss, R. S. The fund of sociability. *Transaction*, 1969, 36-43.

Weiss, R. S. Materials for a theory of social relationships. In W. Bennis et al. (Eds.), *Interpersonal dynamics*. Homewood, Ill.: The Dorsey Press, 1968.

Young, M. & Willmott, P. *Family and kinship in East London*. London: Routeledge & Kegan Paul, 1957.

2

An Approach to Preventive Psychiatry*

During the last few years a number of psychiatrists in different parts of the world have been exploring a new approach to the problem of preventing psychiatric illness. Instead of basing their methods solely, as in the past, on the concept of early casefinding, diagnosis, and treatment, with the goal of circumventing by rapid and radical methods of therapy cases of incipient disease, these workers have set themselves the additional goal of dealing on a community-wide basis with factors which are thought to be pathogenic, with the hope that this will lead to a reduction in the incidence of psychiatric illness in the population.

This approach is complicated by the fact that while we have, as yet, no sure knowledge of the factors which lead to psychiatric pathology, we do know that in any individual case not one but many complicated interrelated factors based on constitution, early childhood experiences, vicissitudes of instinct development, and later sociocultural pressures are responsible for the psychopathological resolution. Our lack of knowledge in regard to the significance of the different factors has to be remedied by continuation of existing research into etiology, but meanwhile

*Lecture delivered in 1954

41

preventive psychiatrists have been able to learn a lesson from their public health colleagues in regard to handling the problem of the multifactorial nature of the picture.

The incidence of cases of clinical tuberculosis, for example, in any community is no longer conceived of in public health circles as merely dependent on the single factor of the presence or absence of the tubercle bacillus. It is recognized that there are many complicated issues involving virulence of the germ, host susceptibility, and various environmental features which will determine whether a particular person exposed to the germ will contract the clinical disease. Many of these factors are either unknown or not easily ascertainable in a community, but this does not prevent the public health man from being able to plan and carry out very effective control programs to reduce clinical tuberculosis in his area—and a good proportion of his program is not focused on the attempt to eradicate the tubercle bacillus itself. The fundamental principle on which he operates is to conceive of the human community as living in an ecological equilibrium with the community of tubercle bacilli, and then attempting to move this equilibrium in a healthy direction, as far as the people are concerned, by dealing with those forces which are accessible to his manipulation. By altering a *significant proportion* of the forces he swings the whole equilibrium over to the "healthy" side.

A similar approach governs some of the recent attempts in community oriented preventive psychiatry. Whether it will have as happy an outcome in the field of mental health as has been achieved by our public health colleagues in the field of physical health remains to be seen. At the moment we are still in the stage of the earliest fumbling attempts; but a discussion of some of these is valuable.

In pursuit of the goal of altering what we think are

unhealthy forces in a community (from the point of view of the mental health, either present or future, of the population) we have been operating in two main ways, which I will call *administrative action* and *personal interaction*. By describing a few examples of procedures which can be classified in this manner I hope to give some idea of the concrete steps in a program of preventive psychiatry.

Administrative Action

The goal here is to reduce preventable stress, or to provide services to assist people facing stress to healthier problem solving, by means of governmental or other administrative action. The idea is to influence laws, statutes, regulations, and customs to achieve these ends. It is recognized that what is involved here is specific culture change, and since all cultures are to be conceived of as *systems* of interrelated forces we realize we must move cautiously, lest a favorable change in one area lead to unexpected unfavorable side effects in other parts of the system.

Despite this danger, which has not always been clearly borne in mind by those of us who have engaged in this type of work, we have, during the past few years, built up a body of experience which indicates that this is a promising avenue for exploration.

The role of the psychiatrist in this type of work is to act as the consultant and advisor to administrative and governmental bodies. He seeks to introduce a point of view to the administrators which is dependent upon his own specialized knowledge of interpersonal forces, and in particular on his knowledge of the psychological needs of individuals and groups. His goal is that the emerging plans or regulations will pay some attention to the mental health needs of the total community and will not add to their mental health burdens.

One example of this work comes from England. This is Bowlby's work on the pathogenic influence of prolonged mother-child separation in early childhood on the child's personality development. He has not yet proved his case, but many of us with clinical experience in this field agree that, other things being equal, prolonged separation of mother and child is not a good thing. The interesting point is that even before he has proved his case, and certainly before he has teased out more than a small proportion of the interrelated forces involved, he has been able to influence the policy of the British Ministry of Health, so that one source of mother-child separation has been radically reduced over the whole country. In 1952, a directive was issued by the Ministry to all hospitals with children's departments to the effect that, wherever possible, daily visiting of children by their parents was to be permitted and encouraged. Latest figures show that at the present time 80% of children's hospitals are carrying out this regulation. A revolutionary blow for the cause of mental health in childhood was struck by that regulation. It is too early to see what the side effects have been in regard to compensatory forces set up among the nurses and the administrators of children's institutions. These will certainly have to be carefully watched; but during the three years following the directive the incidence of mother-child separation in England has been drastically reduced.

Another example comes from Israel. When I first went there in 1948, there was a tremendous wave of immigration. For many reasons the immigrants were housed on arrival in huge camps in large army-style barrack huts. Each hut housed 30-50 people. There were no provisions for privacy, no segregation of family units, and minimal facilities for work. Food was provided in communal dining halls. The immigrants stayed in these huge camps for many months until provision could be made for them to be transferred to permanent settlements. By that time many of them had sunk into an apathetic, dependent state; and when the opportunity for independence and self-respecting work arrived many could not grasp it. As a result partly of mental health consultation as well as of various other complicated changes, the style of reception camps was then radically changed. Newcomers were sent straight from the boat to small temporary encampments dotted about the countryside and often exposed to Arab attacks. They were housed as family units—at first only in canvas tents and later in crude aluminum huts. These were not as cool in summer or as watertight in winter as the big army barrack huts, but they protected the integrity of the family and its strength. Communal kitchens were not provided. Each family had to fend for itself and from the first day they were given productive work to do—difficult work, cleaning rocky hillsides, or draining swamps—but work which fostered their feelings of independence and gave them immediately the feel of being involved in a collaborative endeavor to build a homeland.

Naturally, there were complaints on the part of immigrants who were frightened by the isolation, the physical danger, and the hard work, but the old apathy and overdependence disappeared.

Another example can be cited from Boston, not of successful action, but of the need for action of this type. Across the street from the Whittier Street Health Center in Roxbury is a large new housing project. Since it has been set up there has been a steady drain on the budget of the City of Boston Health Department for the repair of broken windows in the Health Center building. There have been many other indications in the surrounding neighborhood of increasing destructive and delinquent acts by children of various ages. The topic of juvenile delinquency is very complicated and I do not intend to discuss it here, but one or two factors in relation to the housing project are, I believe, not insignificant. Firstly about 50-60% of the families in the project are broken families of one sort or another—either the mother never had a husband, or he left her, or it is a common-law marriage in uneasy equilibrium. The project population contains many other examples of social pathology. There appears to be a diffusion of culture from the unhealthy families to previously healthy ones. Some normal children from healthy families, after living a short time in the project join the delinquent gangs, the core of which is probably made up of the children from the disordered families.

If we ask how does it happen that so high a proportion of the inhabitants are social deviants we find that to get into such a project you have to be on a priority list, where your position depends on a point system. This is determined largely by social need, so that the greater the social pathology the more likely the family is to get to the top of the list. Moreover, administrative pressures are involved, and social agencies are able to apply more pressure on behalf of their clients than individual families can on their own.

It is unfortunate that a psychiatrist was not present while the priority system was being worked out, in order to try and influence the administrators to plan some kind of balanced population for the project. Of course, research is needed to determine what the critical proportion is above which a housing project population cannot accept broken families without endangering its total culture and morals.

Even apart from such research there are one or two

other rather obvious issues on which a psychiatrist might have been able to influence the planners. This project was built with no facilities whatever for the recreation of the children. They have been all collected into one large concentration and given nothing constructive to do. Also the project does not have a custodian or janitor; presumably this role is thought to be appropriate only in higher-class apartment houses. Nobody is, therefore, responsible for the cleanliness of the building, with predictable results.

I have chosen these three examples to illustrate one type of administrative action for preventive psychiatry, the goal being the reduction of the incidence of stress situations or the increase in the provision for the satisfaction of psychological needs. We have to realize, however, that we can never aim at removing *all* problems from the world or ensuring that *all* people are satisfied. We *can* help community leaders arrange facilities so that people who are faced by inevitable stress situations are helped to solve their problems in a healthy way.

There is a good deal of justification for thinking that the capacity for reality-based problem solving is an excellent measure of the mental health of an individual or a group, and also for thinking that the way they handle any significant stress situation in a crisis will have far reaching effects on their future mental health. As a matter of fact, a good deal of the structure of a society can be understood in terms of its purpose in supporting individual members in their solution of life problems. All communities have specialized agencies and individuals who can be conceived of as "caretaking agents," whose function it is to help people in various predicaments. These predicaments, such as birth, death, change of marital and other status, illness, or change of occupation, are normally not conceived of by administrators as mental health crises, and primarily they are not. But community arrangements, such as agency structure and policy, will often affect in no small measure how individuals in these predicaments handle their problems, and what the mental health consequences will be. How a given community deploys its limited caretaking resources may depend on all kinds of social and political factors, but there is room in such planning for a psychiatric consultant who will advise on the effects of policies on the mental health of the population.

Let us take as an example the crisis of having a baby. In the United States, most communities provide prenatal clinics for checking the pregnant woman's physical state, obstetric hospitals for helping her give birth, and well-baby clinics for continued supervision of mother and infant. There is often a domiciliary nursing service, such as a Visiting Nurse Association, which visits the home a few times during pregnancy and once after delivery to supervise the woman's health. Many localities have a municipal health department which provides nurses who make one visit after the mother returns home from the lying-in hospital to check the baby's condition and invite the mother to the well-baby clinic. All or most of these agencies operate separately, with little or no relationship with each other. This may not be ideal policy from the point of view of the physical health of mother and baby, but from the point of view of helping this mother handle the mental health crises of this crucial period it couldn't be worse. A recent experiment conducted by Harvard School of Public Health at Boston Lying-In Hospital has shown the benefit to the developing mother-child and general family relationships of continuity of agency service throughout this period, based upon the fact that there is continuous support to the mother by means of the building up of a stable relationship, as well as the possibility of predicting problems which can be stopped as soon as they start rather than let to run on until they become serious.

Moreover, it is found that one of the most difficult times for the mother is during the three to four weeks after she leaves the lying-in hospital. In most places this is a hiatus as far as agency service is concerned. She is usually expected to make her first visit to the well-baby clinic when the infant is about one month old. During that month she is left largely to her own resources. A change of agency pattern suggested by the above work is intensive domiciliary supervision in certain cases during that period, and earlier contact with the well-baby clinic.

This matter has been found to be of even more importance if there is something wrong with the baby such as a congenital anomaly, not an uncommon happening, as 2% of babies are born with some degree of congenital anomaly. The baby may be very adequately cared-for as regards its physical condition in the hospital, but crippled children's services, for example, do not come into action for many months or longer after the parents have had to deal unaided with the complicated emotional burden of adapting to the child's abnormality. How much time and wasted professional energy would be saved, not to mention avoidable unhappiness and personality distortions for family and child, if community leaders were to realize that a baby with a congenital anomaly represents a situation requiring emergency agency attention concentrated and deployed at the critical period during the first months after birth.

The type of caretaking personnel available in various agencies is also a matter which has preventive psychiatric implications. If a community can afford a certain number of psychiatrists and psychiatric social workers, should these all be operating in remedial institutions, or should some of them be made available to work, for example, in agencies which deal with the ordinary woman having a baby? What are the needs for psychiatric assistance of an agency which is set up to help women who have babies with congenital anomalies?

Such questions point up one of the major difficulties facing a psychiatrist operating within a governmental or other executive group. He must avoid taking on the role of an administrator himself and avoid giving advice based upon his own individual, professional or political vested interests. I would not advocate government by psychiatrists! Moreover, our present psychiatric knowledge about most of the practical issues which come up for administrative consideration is woefully inadequate. The psychiatrist will rarely be in a position to press for some specific administrative action on grounds of scientific knowledge. His role is rather to put what knowledge he has at the disposal of the administrators and to avoid taking over their executive responsibility, either because of his own needs, or because they try and jockey him into doing so.

This leads me to the third aspect of work in this area, which has to be classified on the borderline between administrative action and personal interaction. Although the main goals of the psychiatrist's work in a governing agency are administrative, he achieves these goals by personal interaction with the administrators, and his policies and techniques will be based upon principles which really belong in the next section. He has to gain entry and acceptance in government, and he has to operate in a professional manner in his relationships with his administrative colleagues. His success will depend as much, if not more, on the way he deals with the interpersonal transactions in the building as on the content of any specific advice he may give or psychological information he may impart. An important part of his functioning will relate to helping his colleagues handle the problems of their governing and of their own staff interrelations in as reality-based a way as possible. This does not mean that he should arrogate to himself or allow himself to be put into the role of psychotherapist to his colleagues, but it does mean that he can operate as an expert in the field of inter-personal relations and help, when asked, reduce percep-tual distortions which increase interpersonal tensions. His own professional training has equipped him with a special ability to accept his own human reactions. He can pass some of this benefit on to his colleagues. We do know that this may play an important role in promoting the mental health of the community because of the close rela-tionship which has been shown to exist between the pres-ence or absence of tension in an administrative staff and parallel reactions among the administered population.

This leads to the last point in the present section. A psychiatrist in government will often be asked by the administrators he is assisting to place his knowledge of human beings and techniques of handling them at their disposal for political ends. This is a tricky subject, but there is one positive aspect of it which certainly most psychiatrists would accept. They can advise on relation-ships with the public and ways of achieving those which will be most supportive, and most conducive to adequate problem solving. For instance, they can draw attention to the importance of adequate and uninterrupted channels of communication between administration and population, they can advise on the training and supervision of civil servants in regard to the civility of their service, and they can help tease apart the organizational pressures which might lead to difficulties in this area. They can advise on the probable significance to the people of the content of government communications, and, in short, they can be consultants on morale, though once again policy in these matters will ultimately depend on political and leadership

factors which are outside the province of the mental
health expert.

Personal Interaction

This category of preventive intervention refers to attempts
to change the emotional forces in a person's environment
or the way he solves his life problems, by direct interaction with him or with the people around him. It makes
use more obviously of skills and insights which psychiatrists have developed in their clinical work with patients,
and many of the techniques are clearly modifications of
psychotherapeutic methods, which they resemble more
than they do educational techniques.

It resembles administrative action in that the strategic
goals relate to planning for the reduction of emotional ill
health in the community as a whole, and the greatest good
for the greatest number implies a framework of action in
which economy of effort is a prime consideration. It differs
from administrative action in that the tactics in any
instance are related to personal face-to-face contact with
individuals or small groups. The goals are based upon a
theory of etiology which appears reasonable to us at the
present time. This theory holds that among the significant
factors which will determine the mental health of an
individual are those relating to his emotional milieu, with
special reference to the quality of interpersonal relationships which obtain between certain significant people in
his immediate environment and himself. This is especially
marked in his childhood, and the influence of his parents'
relationships upon the pattern of unfolding of his personality development is well recognized; but it is also found
in his adult life, when the adequate gratification of his
needs and the degree to which he will be supported in

times of stress will depend, among other things, upon the relationships of his family, friends, and work groups.

Allowing for what I have already said in regard to the multifactorial nature of the system in any case, a possible approach to a preventive program might usefully be designed to improve interpersonal relationships or to remedy disordered relationships, rather than waiting for the effect of the latter to lead to psychiatric pathology.

Stated like this, the goal is too broad for effective action; but clinical experience shows us that the scope of the problem can be narrowed down, because there exist in a community certain key individuals who are especially significant for a number of people by reason of their position in the role structure. When one of these key individuals has disordered relationships he may affect the mental health of many people who are dependent upon him. He himself, may or may not show overt signs of psychiatric illness, but he has an obvious noxious effect on the people around him. The analogy of the carrier of an infectious disease such as typhoid comes readily to mind.

The practical question for a preventive program in any community is then to see whether such carriers of mental ill health can be detected, and if so whether their number is such that they can be dealt with; and if techniques can be worked out for improving their interpersonal relationships by methods which are economical enough in time and skilled manpower to allow of community coverage.

This was the kind of formulation we originally made in Jerusalem in 1949. It has undergone fairly extensive development since that time. A brief description of the practical steps we took to implement such a plan follows. We chose mothers of infants as our key people, based on the clinical experience that one mother with certain types of disordered relationships might have a pathogenic effect successively on several of her children. Moreover, our work in child guidance clinics had led us to suppose that we could define and identify the signs of disordered mother-child relationships which would mark any particular mother a carrier or not—realizing, of course, that a particular mother would have idiosyncratic relationships with each of her children, but hypothesizing that many who showed a pathogenic relationship to one child would have a spread to others.

We then hunted in the community for these carriers. We narrowed our search down by focusing on well-baby clinics, where there is a high concentration of mothers of infants; and we developed rapid screening devices for scanning the total population of mothers in each clinic. We found about 10% of mothers were screened out as having undoubted or probable disorders of relationship with their infants. We then worked out techniques for motivating these mothers to cooperate in a deeper investigation of their relationships; where the original suspicion was found to be valid, we developed techniques of involving the mother in a treatment relationship. The next step in the process was critical: could we find methods of ameliorating the disordered relationships which would be economical? If the disorder were based on some neurosis of the mother, and all we had achieved was a list of candidates for adult psychotherapy, we wouldn't be much better off from the community point of view than if we had waited until the infant grew into a child with psychiatric symptoms, and then treated it as a psychiatric patient. There would be some gain, but not enough.

We feel that one of the triumphs of this work has been that we did manage to work out techniques of "unlinking" the child from the mother's intrapsychic disorder or, in other words, of improving the mother's relationships with this and her other children without having to become committed to undertaking the often major task of treating her core problems by lengthy methods of psychotherapy. We developed techniques of focused or segmental case-work or psychotherapy which concentrated on the *inter-personal* problem of the mother and in most cases did not encroach more than a minimum amount on her *intraper-sonal* problem. We found that in the majority of cases such techniques were possible because the disorder in relationships was involved only in one segment or sector of the range of emotional problems which had been crys-tallized in the personality pattern of that mother.

This research is still being continued in Jerusalem. It will take several years before many of the loose ends can be tied up with any pretense at scientific validity. But meanwhile the impressions gained are that it is certainly practical to go into a community and identify a major proportion of those mothers who have pathogenic relation-ships to their infants, and it is possible to think in practical terms of deploying sufficient skilled staff to remedy these disorders and achieve community coverage. The average number of sessions per case with the present technique was about eight to ten. Group techniques could probably be developed to make such a plan even more practical from the community point of view. But both the individual and the group techniques demand a staff of experienced and highly trained psychiatric workers, which is not likely to be available except in a few privileged com-munities.

Moreover, since 1949, we have become a bit more sophisticated about analyzing the field of forces in a per-son's emotional milieu, and we can no longer think with-out discomfort of isolating mother-child relationships in as static a way as we did then. For instance, we were im-pressed in Jerusalem by the fact that in certain cases we benefited the mother-child relationships and the follow-up investigation showed a subsequent, and maybe consequent, disturbance of wife-husband relationships, or some other more subtle alteration of the field of forces in the family. Even for the original infant, when he had developed past the stage of almost complete dependence on his mother, the change in family equilibrium which resulted from the original unlinking maneouver was sometimes as productive of psychiatric disturbance as the original situation could have been.

Another relevant consideration was the idea that we might track down the factors which lead to disordered mother-child relationships, and that dealing with these might be easier than the highly skilled job of segmental casework. It might be easy enough so that it could be entrusted to public health workers who had had no lengthy psychiatric training. This hope was spurred on by the discovery that certain traumatic events during pregnancy, such as a failed attempt at abortion, or the death or injury of another child, often led to especially pathogenic types of disorders of the future mother-child relationship; and such cases could often be easily cured by public health nurses or obstetricians who were alerted to the special mental health significance of such traumatic events and equipped with mental health first-aid techniques, such as methods for reducing excessive conscious or preconscious guilt.

Such thinking then highlighted the significance of certain experiences in Jerusalem and similar experiences in Boston, where Erich Lindemann had been working on the manifestations of the bereavement process in adults and its relationship to the subsequent development of various psychiatric disorders. The concept that emerged was one which has been familiar to lay people, to novelists and to dramatists for centuries but has till now received scant attention from psychiatrists—namely the importance of periods of crisis in determining individual and group development. Such a crisis is provoked when someone faces an obstacle to important life goals, which is, for a time, insurmountable through the utilization of customary methods of problem solving. A period of disorganization ensues, during which many different abortive attempts at solution are attempted. Eventually some kind of adaptation is achieved, which may or may not be in the best interests of that person and his fellows.

The important point for the development of our present theme is that disturbances of interpersonal relationships between mothers and children and also within the total field of forces in a family can often be seen clinically to originate during a certain crisis period, and can be conceived of as one type of maladaptive solution of the crisis problem—a vicarious solution by projection and displacement at the emotional expense of someone within the family orbit. In an oversimplified way we can say the crisis was resolved by means of the development of the disordered relationship.

Such thinking led to the research project which was conducted at the Whittier Street Family Guidance Center. A number of categories of commonly occurring stress were chosen, such as birth of a premature baby, or a baby with a congenital anomaly, or the diagnosis of tuberculosis in a family member. Families who are in crises as a result of these problems were then studied, with the intention of describing the range of adaptive and maladaptive responses. The hope was that it will be possible to separate at one end of the spectrum those families who solve the crisis problems by developing disordered relationships.

It is further hoped that in the same way that Lindemann, by his study of normal grief work in bereavement, can now help to steer back onto the adaptive path those bereaved persons who show signs of deviating, the present study will equip us with specific information to help families in crisis. I would emphasize that such techniques are of a first-aid variety—they require little time and not too much training—since they handle mainly preconscious mechanisms. In other words, they would be available for widespread use in a public health setting, and such a service would make use of psychiatric personnel only in a consultative or advisory role.

This leads me to my last point, a consideration of possibly the most important type of preventive psychiatric activity which comes under the heading of personal interaction: mental health consultation.

I referred previously to key people who exert a potent effect on the mental health of a number of other individuals. When we first thought of this concept we had in mind blood relations, close friends or people occupying special roles in a person's work or recreational group, but it became rapidly obvious that in a community there existed a network of institutional roles which fitted into this category—namely people like nurses, doctors, clergymen, teachers, or policemen. These are the "caretaking agents" of the community. At particular times they are certainly key people in affecting the mental health of many others. It is significant that these particular times are usually times of crisis for their clients.

A school teacher, for example, is of importance to the educational progress of her pupils. To some extent she is of importance to their mental health, according to the general type of interpersonal relationships she manifests and the consequent emotional atmosphere she builds up in her classroom. But her importance as a factor in the emotional life of some particular pupil suddenly increases tremendously if that pupil is faced by a crisis problem. At that time the supportive or unhelpful activities of the teacher may be instrumental in tipping the child towards or away from a healthy adaptive solution of his life problems. The same situation can be seen to hold with a clergyman, and even more so with a nurse or doctor. The quality of care which they are able to deliver when an individual or a family is in crisis may be a crucial factor in determining the outcome as far as the future mental health of their clients is concerned.

Each of these professional caretaking groups has its own subculture—its own traditional ways of perceiving its clients' problems and of handling them. We can think in terms of their having a "professional persona," a fairly standardized range of ways of handling their professional problems, including the usual human reactions of clients who are in crisis. This range is usually flexible and allows for individual variation according to the idiosyncratic personality structure of the individual professional worker.

Two points interest us in regard to this. First, are the traditional ways of helping people, in line with the professional persona, effective from the mental health point of view? We have to realize that the primary purpose of the professional persona is not the pursuit of mental health but the specific goals of that profession—teaching, doctoring, and so on. If they are not effective for mental health, can we work out ways of making them more effective, ways which are compatible with the primary goals and the general framework of that profession? There is no good in trying to make nurses into little psychiatrists; even if we succeeded, we would then need to look for people to train as nurses. What is needed is a study of what the range of operations is in the different professions, plus a good deal more research along Whittier Street lines to provide specific information about the most helpful behavior by care-taking agents during crisis periods.

Secondly, how do individual personality factors interfere with the professional persona, and what can be done to prevent either generalized disorders of interpersonal functioning or specific upsets in the caretaking agent from interfering with his capacity to help his clients in crisis? This is a subject on which we have done a lot of work, and *I* can only refer very briefly to it here.

Working mainly in educational institutions both here and in Israel, we have found that the specific features of a child's symptoms or his life situation at the moment may be such that they stimulate unsolved problems in the teacher. The latter then, instead of helping the child in his difficulties, actually hinders him from finding an adaptive solution. In other cases the child's crisis is actually precipitated as a direct reaction to some intrapersonal problem of the teacher or some disequilibrium in the social structure of the school or in its relationship with the surrounding community. There is always some special consonance of the life situation of the child and the characteristics of the field situation which accounts for the linkage. Different children are used vicariously at different times as symptoms of the segmental disorder of teacher or school at that time.

In order to deal with this problem a special technique of mental health consultation has been worked out, which has now reached the stage that its theoretical structure and practical methodology can be put down on paper and can be taught systematically to trainees. The mental health consultant visits various schools in his area and offers to discuss "problem children" with the teachers. In any school most of the cases referred involve a child in a state of crisis and one or more members of the teaching staff also in crisis. The child may have some quite objective illness, but usually he is referred because his trouble and that of the teacher have become linked. The teacher characteristically displaces his own problems almost entirely onto those of the child, and the consultant in his discussions accepts this displacement. They both discuss the child's problems, but the consultant remains continually aware of the possible implications to the teacher and the institution of the details of this discussion. He does not interfere with the teacher's defense mechanisms, but within their framework he tries to release some of the tension deriving from the underlying problem. This reduction of tension allows the teacher to dissipate his stereotyped perception of the child, who can then be perceived as a *child with problems* rather than a *problem child.* The teacher is then assisted to help the child in his human predicament, and since the details of this have a special significance for himself this has a reflexive effect on his own segmental problem.

A successful series of consultations—usually three or four sessions are needed to help a teacher deal with a crisis—assists not only the particular child referred, but often has a radical effect on one of the segments of that teacher's problems which has been interfering with his professional functioning. This means that future children with the same problem will probably not tip him into crisis, and he will be able to help them find an adaptive solution to their problems within the framework of his role as a teacher.

This type of technique provides a small number of highly trained psychiatric workers with a tool for working, through the intermediation of a large number of community caretaking agents, with a very large number of members of the population at periods of crucial importance to their future mental health. The results still remain to be validated. They seem reasonably good so far, but if this technique doesn't turn out to be what we want, we must search for others which will achieve similar goals.

3

How to Detect the Early Stages of Mental Disturbance in Children*

We are living in an era of prevention in our approach to physical illness. Much of our success in the public health field comes from the detection of early cases of disease on a community-wide basis, so that treatment can be both short and effective in interrupting the development of major illness. What is more logical than the idea of copying this process in the field of mental health? It is appealing to consider application of this model to the problem of handling the mental disturbances of childhood, since there is plenty of evidence that, if not adequately treated, many emotional disorders of the child persist into adult life; or else they act as precursors of future adult breakdown by leaving weakness in the foundations of the personality which increase vulnerability to later stress.

If we could provide an answer to the question of how to detect the early stages of mental disturbance in children, and if we could disseminate this knowledge to appropriate people throughout the community—to physicians, nurses, kindergarteners, school teachers, and last but not least to parents—we might be able to make arrangements for children with early disturbances to receive

*Opening lecture at Mental Health Institute, St. Croix, Virgin Islands, January 26, 1957.

prompt treatment; with a minimum expenditure of professional effort, we would be well on the way to ridding our communities of the blight of mental illness.

The big obstacle to this plan, however, is the apparent lack of an answer to this central question of early detection. As a professor of public health mental health and as an experienced child psychiatrist, I have no clear answer to this question, nor am I familiar with any other expert in this field who has one.

Obstacles to Finding the Best Means of Detection

The first problem I meet in trying to find an answer is that few, if any, mental disturbances in childhood—or among adults for that matter—take the form of circumscribed disease entities (for example, measles, chickenpox, or typhoid fever) in which the illness has a fairly typical and characteristic clinical picture. There are undoubtedly many variations in the history, course, and outcome of such illnesses, but however much the physical configuration and makeup of two individuals may differ, the signs and symptoms when they contract measles will be very similar, and will be quite different from the clinical picture each will show when he gets chickenpox.

The very words we use in describing the process attest to the significance of what is happening. We talk of *individuals* contracting a specific disease. We can describe that disease in terms of the agents which are essential in its causation, such as bacteria or viruses; in terms of certain metabolic changes in the chemical functioning of certain bodily cells, which to a lesser or greater degree invariably accompany the disease process; and in terms of more gross alterations in the structure and functioning of bodily organs, which underly the characteristic signs and symptoms by which the physician recognizes the illness. It is a relatively simple matter to observe the course of development of many examples of each illness of this type and to describe a characteristic clinical history, starting with the prodromal and early signs and symptoms which occur in certain specific describable sets of circumstances and then developing through definite stages to the main pathological picture. It is also possible to collect and describe examples of minimal or abortive illness in which the developmental process becomes arrested for a variety of causes before the major disease picture is reached.

A few of the mental disturbances of childhood seem to fit into this model. Most of these are on the borderline between physical illness and mental illness, like cerebral palsy, which is due to brain damage during the birth process; mongolism or other mental deficiencies associated with congenital abnormalities of neurological or metabolic development and the upsets in mental development associated with damage to the brain by accident or disease during childhood. The diagnosis of such conditions, especially when they are mild, during the first weeks or months of a baby's life, may occasionally tax the efforts of a pediatrician, but this is in essence as simple a problem as the detection of the earliest signs of measles or typhoid. It need not concern us here, as these conditions form only a tiny proportion of our problem and are quite untypical of the rest.

It is when we turn our attention to the main body of mental disorders in childhood that our problems really begin, because these do not lend themselves at all to being described along the lines of the model we have been discussing up to now. In the fully developed disturbance, the child may certainly complain of clinical symptoms of unpleasant or unwelcome feelings, and he may manifest clinical signs in the form of deviations of behavior and functioning from his previous state or from an ideal norm; but although some of these signs and symptoms may be similar to what we may see in other sick children, the disorder as a whole—in its history, type of onset, course, and outcome—is usually a development of the idiosyncratic functioning of that individual child. It is to be thought of as a *reaction* of the child, and not as an *illness* which he has "contracted." So although we can classify, in a rough kind of way, certain commonly occurring characteristic types of reactions of different children, and give them specific names (such as anxiety state, hysteria, behavior disorder, personality disorder, or neurosis), we are not really able to specify and delimit the psychological deviations of a particular child—beyond saying that at the time we examined him he appeared to be behaving in such and such a way. Any assumption, either of cause or of outcome, which would be based upon the label we applied to his behavior would be most unreliable. If we really wished to answer the questions "why is he like this?" and "what will he become?", we must not study his signs and symptoms, which may be classified as fitting one of these reaction types, but we must study the child as an individual, with an idiosyncratic history, a certain constitutional makeup, and temperament, all of which have been interacting during his lifetime with the forces of his physical and emotional environment, with his mother and father and siblings, with his playmates, his schoolteachers, and his religious group. We will wish to study what problems he has faced during his lifetime and how he has solved them, and we will wish to pay special attention to the range of problem-solving skills he has developed, with special reference to certain types of problems, the solutions of which have made undue demands upon his emotional or intellectual resources.

In other words, many of the kind of questions which

could be simply answered in a case of measles merely by defining it as a case of that illness, could only, in the case of a typical childhood emotional disorder, be answered by an intensive and complicated study of the individual's innermost mental functioning, and not solely from the label we might apply to his clinical picture.

Mental Disturbance and Normal Functioning

Mental disturbance is not an alien process which has its own characteristic appearance and history, and which is superimposed upon the ordinary functioning of the child, but is an alteration of the child's usual functioning resulting from his attempts to solve current and former life problems.

The implication of this for our present discussion is clear. We cannot expect to be able to make lists of those signs and symptoms which occur universally in children as the early manifestations of certain mental disturbances; any particular item of disturbed behavior will have a different meaning from one child to the next, and must be understood not in relation to a circumscribed disease process but in relation to the adaptive responses of a particular individual person in a particular situation. Bed-wetting, for example, will have a quite different significance from one child to the next. In one it may represent anxiety at the imagined threat of loss of parental love on the occasion of the birth of a sibling; in another it may be a manifestation of rebelliousness against a father made irritable and punitive by business worries; in a third it may be a reaction to the loss of the mother due to death or illness; and in a fourth it may be associated with temporary difficulties in adapting to a new school.

It may be argued, however, that whatever its individual

cause may be, bedwetting is *per se* to be regarded as a sign of mental disturbance in the same way that a rise of temperature is a nonspecific sign of bodily disturbance. This is true to an extent, but if we are trying to detect the early stages of the type of mental disturbances which would require psychiatric treatment and in the absence of which there would be serious incapacity and suffering, the identification of bedwetting cannot be of much direct value to us. In all the instances previously cited, for example, the symptom may spontaneously clear up after a few days, weeks, or months, and no mental disturbance may result. On the other hand, different children exposed to roughly similar circumstances, who do not react with bedwetting but with some other behavioral deviation—or, to make matters more complicated, with no externally obvious change in behavior—may later turn out to be suffering from mental disturbances whose origin can be retrospectively traced back to that particular time.

Our difficulties are further compounded by the knowledge that if we make a list of what might be predictive signs and symptoms—temper tantrums, sleep disturbances, feeding disturbances, nail biting, masturbation, overactivity, underactivity, stealing, aggressive outbursts, excessive jealousy, failure at school, truanting, nightmares, phobias, and so on—we find that practically no child gets through the period of childhood without suffering some time from at least one of them. Moreover, we are not helped by adding up all the symptoms which a particular child manifests over a period and expecting that if the number exceeds a certain threshold this means he is a "nervous" child and will later turn out to develop a neurosis, a personality disorder, or some other form of mental disturbance. Certainly by the time he has such a disturbance he will probably show a number of these symptoms, but other children who have a greater number of symptoms will be found, on examination, *not* to be suffering currently or subsequently from mental disturbances.

How then can we ever say that a certain child is suffering from a fully developed mental disturbance? The answer to this is that a specialist's investigation of the child's behavior in his interaction with his environment will demonstrate a consistent inability to function at a level consonant with the expectable stages of his mental development. His functioning in the various areas of his life field must be scrutinized, and the intrapsychic configuration of his personality must be assessed by psychiatric interview techniques and psychological testing. Child psychiatry has advanced sufficiently for us to obtain reliable results from such an investigation conducted by well-trained workers; in this discussion I am theoretically relying upon such a procedure to validate any statement I make about the presence or absence of mental disturbance in connection with the determination of whether any particular set of symptoms does or does not succeed in predicting its subsequent appearance.

Flexibility of Personality and Child Development

To return for a moment to my previous statement that "nervous" symptoms are so common in normal children that they cannot be relied upon as predictors of mental disturbance: The reason this is so relates to the main characteristic of psychological functioning in childhood, namely the flexibility and plasticity, and what might be called lability, of the child's personality. A child is not a little adult; his mind is not like a miniature adult's mind, as perhaps his body appears. A child's personality starts off at birth in a quite undifferentiated state, and develops by a series of stages into that of the mature adult. Each of these stages is qualitatively different from the previous and subsequent ones, and personality development proceeds through a series of transitions from one stage to the next, as a result of a complicated series of interactions between the child and his environment. In order to grow and develop in this way the child's personality must remain labile and plastic, and rigid patterns of behavior are hardly to be expected. Moreover, it is impossible to conceive that this complicated development involving the interconnections of so many forces, physical, cultural, and social, could ever take place without the occasional building up of organismic tensions or frictions between child and environment due to his needs not being fulfilled or his inability to fulfill demands made upon him. When such tensions build up, there have to be avenues for discharge, and the various symptoms and behavioral irregularities we have already mentioned fulfill this purpose exactly. Most of them are commonly used by children as safety valves to maintain their mental balance; such safety valves are often needed, especially during important transitional phases of development.

Since we now know quite a lot about the sequence of developmental stages in the growth of a child's personality, might this not be useful in detecting signs of faulty development which might be due to the beginnings of a mental disturbance? For example, if we know that children normally achieve a particular stage of development by a certain age, could we not try to identify those children of that age who do not show such development, and use this as a method of predicting mental disorder? This approach has certainly been tried, but does not work very well as a method of prediction; although a general timetable of development can be drawn up, there are too many exceptions for retardation to be acceptable as a predictive device. In other words, some children develop more slowly than average and may have special difficulty in moving from one particular stage to the next, and yet by the time they reach maturity they seem mentally healthy. Other children, by contrast, who are found to be emotionally ill, have developed in perfect line with the timetable, at least until their disordered functionings interfered with various important aspects of their lives as a whole, including the development of their personalities. This means that screening a population of children for those with a lag in development will screen out a number of healthy children who are, by nature or by nurture, slower than average; also, such a sample will also include some children who are, or in the past have been, suffering from a psychological disorder. The latter, however, will not usually be in its early stages if it has already interfered in any significant way with personality development.

Regression

While on the topic of the timetable of development of the child's personality, I would like to discuss the mechanism of regression, which is a common phenomenon contributing to the ubiquity of behavioral deviations in childhood. The very lability of the psychological functioning which allows the child's personality to develop in a forward direction also permits it at times to move backwards to earlier and outmoded patterns of functioning. This usually occurs when the child is having difficulty using the skills appropriate to his current level of development to cope with a present demand. He retires from the reality-obstacle into the fantasy-security of earlier childhood and its remembered comforts. This may result in a dramatic change in his behavior which by its suddenness, and by reason of the inappropriateness of his actions to a child of his age, may be quite alarming to his family and even to the professional worker called in to deal with him. Here again we find that continued contact with these children shows that although some eventually develop mental disturbances, the vast majority regain the ability to act their age fairly quickly and suffer no pathological after-effects.

I don't want to leave this consideration of the timetable of personality development without paying tribute to those research workers who have worked so hard to clarify it for us, since by so doing they have helped us to avoid one pitfall into which many of us used to fall—that of calling a certain behavior pattern "abnormal" which we now realize to be a perfectly usual reaction in a child of that particular age. This is especially so in regard to adolescence.

Benign and Dangerous Behavioral Changes

It might seem by now that as a child psychiatrist I am either not seriously interested at all in behavioral disorders in childhood or that I even welcome them as a sign of a normal growth process, and that I subscribe to the philosophy which says "pay no attention to the child's symptoms and he will grow out of it."

This is an oversimplification. I do not believe we can rely upon these symptoms as our major criteria for predicting mental disorder, but I do not doubt that they do have significance in helping us penetrate the mysteries of childhood development; parents and professional child care workers certainly should never neglect them. They are visible signs that some change is taking place in the child. We expect a child to be changing, but as adults it is our role to keep a watchful eye on this process and to be prepared to be helpful whenever necessary. Child psychiatrists have, in the last few years, collected ample evidence to demonstrate scientifically what ordinary people have always known: The way children develop is dependent on the ways their parents, family, and other key figures in their life—such as educators, physicians, or clergymen—treat them. Unfortunately, the publication of a good deal of this scientific work has done more harm than good, as parents and educators have become anxious and self-conscious in their child rearing roles, and in some cases have begun to feel guilty whenever a child under their care has shown signs of having problems. The slogan has become "mother is the root of all evil," and lately fathers, too, are beginning to be implicated. I will return in a few minutes to this important topic, but before I do I would like to discuss the child care implications of the behavioral deviations I have been talking about.

Whenever a child's behavior changes, I think the responsible adults, whether parents or professional, should ask themselves why this change is taking place. From what I have said so far they should feel some confidence in asking this question without alarm, no matter how dramatic the change in behavior and how out of keeping with former development. It may be that knowledge of the child as a person with his characteristic ways of reacting to problems will quickly provide an answer to the question. For instance, a mother who on previous occasions has observed that her nine-year-old son has reacted with especially marked misery and moping as a response to separation experiences, ever since the age of four when his father was away from home in the army, may quickly think of such an explanation when the boy seems strangely out of sorts and uninterested in his food. On inquiry she may then find that his best friend at school has left town with his parents, or that a favorite teacher has had to go into the hospital for an operation. In another instance a child's reaction may be quite new and unusual, as in the case of a sturdy, independent three-year-old who suddenly started to wet his pants, have temper tantrums, and cling babyishly to his mother. Here the parents have to ask themselves "what is happening at present in the boy's development, or in our family circle, to which he may be reacting?" It is important to realize that a child, and especially a small child, is an integral part of his family and sociocultural environment. People sometimes strangely imagine that a child exists in a vacuum, and sometimes they appear to believe that he is deaf and blind to all that goes on around him. In fact, we are coming more and more to realize how sensitive the usual child is to the interpersonal forces which enmesh him. In a family the young child, being the most labile psychosocial organism, may in fact be the first or the only family member to register certain tensions which result from external pressures or intra-family stresses. If the parents think of the child as a possible thermometer of the family temperature, they may quickly identify the cause of his behavior disorder. In our present case the mother may not realize the connection, but when she complains to her physician about her son's strangely babyish behavior, the doctor may remind her that she is 4 months pregnant; this fact, although probably intellectually incomprehensible to the three-year-old, nevertheless has altered the family atmosphere and has preoccupied her, so he feels a cutting down of his emotional supplies and is rebelling against it.

As we investigate case after case of children who exhibit recent symptoms of behavioral disturbance we begin to realize that although the causes sometimes are hidden from us, those which we do clarify show that these children are emitting signals of distress, or are using tension-release mechanisms, as they face problems either primarily within themselves or within their family circle (or, in older children, in their school, social, or religious groups). Children, because of their weakness and inexperience, find many problems very difficult or insoluble. This is not altogether a bad thing; it is helpful for their development that they are exposed to a sufficient number of problems which they can only solve by special effort, so that they are stimulated by the challenge. As a result a child will not infrequently be faced by a problem of importance —one which endangers satisfaction of one of his fundamental needs—when he as yet does not have the learned skill nor the innate strength to solve it satisfactorily within a short time. It may be that by working on his own at the problem, or tackling it with the help of his family, he may eventually solve it. In any case, the impact of the problem will be followed by a lesser or greater period of time when the child will be wrestling with the difficulty under conditions of raised organismic tension, and associated negative feelings of anxiety, frustration, anger, guilt, or shame, according to the detailed meaning of the problem to him. We refer to this period of upset as crisis.

Types of Crisis

In the light of these considerations we get a deeper insight into the meaning of the "nervous symptoms" of childhood and the reasons they are so common. We can classify the causes of these crises, many of which I have already referred to. Some of these crises are primarily *endogenous*, such as those produced by the inevitable transitional stages between successive developmental phases. As the child leaves one organized phase, he must pass through a period of some disorganization before he can achieve the next phase which is organized differently from the last. Some problems which he solved easily in the old manner are difficult or impossible to handle for a while in the transitional period of dedifferentiation until he learns to solve them in a new way by using his more mature approach.

Other types of endogenous crises relate to complicated biopsychological imbalances; as during adolescence, when the hormonal changes of puberty produce increases in instinctual pressures which interfere with the child's relationships with his social environment, and reflexively affect his concept of his own identity with consequent disorganization of his social functioning.

Another major category of crises may be classified as *exogenous*. These can be traced to problems originating primarily in the child's environment, although of course the essential element of crisis is connected with the interpenetration of these factors with the intrapsychic functioning of the child. Among the exogenous varieties may be mentioned those related to tasks or role performance at school, or in the family and social circle, and those related to key interpersonal emotional relationships with parents, siblings, friends, or teachers. Especially important are sudden changes in the demand for role performance, as in transition between kindergarten and school, or junior to high school, and in the pattern of interaction with loved ones or friends, for example, due to the death of a parent or separation from siblings or friends.

In all these circumstances the child's disordered behavior is the sign that he is in crisis and is wrestling with a problem. His period of wrestling may lead to success on some level, or to failure. Whatever the result he will eventually settle down to a new pattern of functioning. It is clear that the period of upset is not to be considered a period of illness, but a natural and expectable period of adaptation during which essential mental work is being done by the child. The details of his symptoms, which are the side effects of the process of struggling with the problem, do not at all enable us to predict the outcome. And it is the nature of this outcome—the type of solution or nonsolution of the problem—which will determine to a greater or lesser degree the future mental health of the child and the adult-to-be.

Context of the Problem

These considerations lead to the suggestion that if we wish to get closer to the answer to the problem of predicting mental disorder in children, we should investigate how they deal with the problems which precipitate these crises. One way of detecting the crises is by taking cognizance of periods of disordered behavior of the type I have discussed. I have already given some brief indication that the crisis problems may be meaningfully classified, and perhaps research will show that the types of solutions may also be described and categorized; thus unhealthy solutions may be identified—that is, those which lead to dissipation of mental energy and to the frustration of basic needs leading to emotional illness. I have also suggested that in appraising this situation it is best to focus not on the child alone, but on the section of society which encompasses the network of human interrelationships of which he is an integral part—usually his family, but as he gets older including also his school and friendship groups. It is in the context of the forces identifiable within this broader focus that the child's problem and the factors influencing its solution will be best seen; and the equilibrium achieved after the crisis is over can best be assessed in regard to the child's future mental health. If this equilibrium represents a stabilized set of harmful environmental and intrapsychic patterns, whether these are or are not accompanied at that time by symptoms in the child, we can infer that his chances of future emotional disorder as a result of recent happenings are high, and appropriate preventive intervention will be indicated.

Case History: The Adams Family

A case example may illustrate some of these points. It is drawn from a study we carried out at Harvard School of Public Health on the responses of families to crisis.

The Adams family was facing a serious problem. Mrs. Adams had been taken into a tuberculosis sanatorium suffering from advanced pulmonary tuberculosis complicated by a tuberculoma of the brain. Mr. Adams remained at home with his two daughters, aged 14 and 12, and his son Jackie, aged 7. He continued at work, and managed the housework when he returned home in the evening with the help of the two girls.

The Adams family had been fairly happy and contented until the mother became ill. They had faced no serious problem in the past. Mrs. Adams had apparently been the dominant person in the family, and her husband played a somewhat subservient and dependent role in the home, although he had a steady work record as the foreman in a dry cleaning establishment.

The housework had been neglected during the previous few months of Mrs. Adams' illness, but during the first six to eight weeks after she went into the hospital the situation became even more upset. Mr. Adams was ineffectual in assuming the leadership role left vacant by his wife's departure, and both he and the girls seemed tense and disorganized. They handled their feelings about Mrs.

Adams' illness and absence from the home in a special way: they didn't talk about it; they pretended that they were not worried about the danger to her life; and they even tried to pretend that they were glad she was out of the house, because of the nuisance she had been during the last few months with her increasing irritability and ineffectuality. Instead of facing their individual and group problem of trying to master their unpleasant feelings of anxiety and depression, they defended themselves against the situation by denial and avoidance.

Little Jackie behaved differently—partly perhaps because, being the youngest and most dependent on the mother, he was hardest hit by her absence, and possibly also because he had not yet developed the capacity to maintain so active a denial of so pressing a problem. He became quite miserable, and cried and whined the whole time, freely verbalizing his longing for his mother and his fears about what the doctors were doing to her.

The reaction of the rest of the family toward him was interesting. They not only did not comfort him as they would probably have done a couple of months earlier, but they in fact all turned on him whenever he complained and told him to "shut his mouth." They called him a "pest" and a "misery," and they began actively to illtreat him.

Mealtimes were very irregular, and most of the time Mr. Adams and the girls ate separately. Jackie's feeding was neglected, and the others became disgusted with him because during this time he began to show signs of gluttony and was continually stealing food. He also began stealing money from the money box of one of his sisters, for which he was repeatedly beaten; he began wandering off from home and truanting from school. Some of his wandering seemed a direct reaction to the general neglect which was his lot in the family circle and to the lack of supervision of his activities. He wandered disconsolately around the neighborhood for hours, and when he didn't come home until late, Mr. Adams and the girls became anxious, and on his return beat him savagely.

In short, Jackie became the black sheep of the family—or, to be more exact, the scapegoat. Mr. Adams put this in a nutshell on one occasion when he said: "In my period of trouble the girls are a bit of a help—they wash the dishes and clean the house—but Jackie's only job is to worry me!" It looked as though all the negative feelings of the father and daughters were being displaced onto the boy, and when their tension rose too high because of their unexpressed feelings about Mrs. Adams' illness and the family predicament, they relieved the tension by attacking Jackie.

Jackie, on his part, reacted in a way that made matters worse, because by talking freely about his longings and fear for his mother he endangered the defenses of the rest of the family who were trying to deny and escape the problem. And he reacted to the rejection and deprivation of family love by delinquent, rebellious acts which still further aggravated his position by infuriating his family.

An interesting aspect of this story which makes it so apt an illustration to this topic is that after Mrs. Adams had been in the sanatorium for about six weeks, her condition took a turn for the worse. For a while her life was despaired of because the tuberculoma burst and she developed tubercular meningitis. This catastrophe proved too much for the family's defenses of denial. Mr. Adams and the girls suddenly realized the full implications of the situation, and their anxiety and depression came out openly. They wept, suffered from insomnia and poor concentration at work, and they became preoccupied with anxious discussions regarding the patient's chances and their own impending bereavement.

Something else happened. They began to comfort and support each other, and strangely enough Mr. Adams now suddenly took on a major leadership role in the family—with his daughters very willingly taking on the role of followers. The home improved its appearance and the household routines, such as mealtimes and bedtimes, became regular.

Most interesting of all, the scapegoating of Jackie suddenly ceased. In his open reactions to his mother's illness he was no longer a deviant; he was taken back completely into the family circle to receive the comfort and love which he needed. The effect of this change in treatment on his behavior was dramatic. He stopped his wandering and his rebellious actions, and although he was clearly still quite miserable about his mother, he now looked like a sad little boy and not like a beaten puppy, as in the past. His stealing did not cease completely, but the mark of the changed family attitude towards him was his father's statement: "When Jackie comes home and feels miserable because his mother is not here, he takes a penny from his sister's box to comfort himself."

This story has a happy ending, because Mrs. Adams responded favorably to a new drug treatment in the sanatorium, eventually recovered, and came home. And little Jackie is now apparently as well off as he has ever been, none the worse for his two-month period of ostracism and deprivation.

This case illustrates very well the central point of this chapter, that an appraisal of Jackie's condition at the height of the crisis would have had little meaning if it had consisted of a list of his numerous subjective symptoms and gross behavioral deviations. It might have led to the erroneous conclusion that he was, or would soon become, a very sick boy.

The child's condition took on more meaning when he

was considered against the background of the family situation, and it was realized that he was struggling not only against the insoluble problem of maternal deprivation, but also against the equally serious problem of family scapegoating. A prediction based even on this evidence would, however, have probably been fallacious, since it too would have pointed to a pathological result. It was not until the crisis had been resolved that the stable outcome could be seen and it could be realized that the scapegoating was a symptom of the family crisis, which represented a temporary safety valve to lower tension until an adaptive solution could be worked out. Our present knowledge of the problem-solving patterns of families in crisis would not have allowed us to predict this outcome at the beginning or at the height of the crisis, and only continued observation of the behavior of the family members eventually allowed us to understand what was transpiring.

It is conceivable that had certain factors been different, this family might never have adapted adequately to Mrs. Adams' illness and the scapegoating of Jackie might have proved a stable end result. In that case it would have been valid for us to predict that his delinquent behavior would have represented the beginnings of a potentially serious emotional disorder, which in the future might well have needed considerable psychiatric treatment.

Interrelationships of Responsible Factors

One final point relates to the question of responsibility for Jackie's symptoms. Should Mr. Adams and his daughters have felt guilty for scapegoating Jackie and not comforting him in his troubles? As a matter of fact, for a time Mr. Adams actively blamed Jackie for being a nuisance.

This was a common attitude up to 20 years ago, when it was customary for parents to feel that children with behavioral disturbance were "bad boys" and "pests." It would seem that by now the climate of opinion has changed so much that in the unlikely event that Mr. Adams were to read this story and were to recognize himself (through the distortions I have introduced to preserve his anonymity) he might feel that he was a very bad father and had been guilty of harming his son.

Of course, this reaction of parental guilt is just as inappropriate as that of blaming the disturbed child. We might as well blame Mrs. Adams, whose illness precipitated the whole difficulty. We might even blame Mr. Adams' father, who presented to his growing son a model of an ineffectual man, partly because he had lost a leg in the war and was a lifelong invalid. Or should we blame the doctors in the sanatorium, who "misguidedly" took such good care of Mrs. Adams that her condition did not deteriorate sufficiently to alter the family's reaction pattern for 6 weeks after her admission?

As we study a case such as this—and although it is a bit more dramatic, it is really not unlike many many others—we realize that responsibility for the development of mental ill health or mental health in a child is the end result of numerous very complicated factors, and it is not possible even to think in terms of simple cause and effect, let alone moral responsibility, blame, and guilt. I am not saying that evil people do not exist in this world, and that some of them do not selfishly exploit their children, but usually these parents do not feel guilty. The ones who do are parents caught in a complicated network of forces—parents who do their best with the resources at their disposal to handle the problems that beset them, and only add to those problems by misguided attempts to oversimplify their situation through allotting blame to themselves or others. Work is needed to clarify the question of how to detect the early signs of mental disorder in childhood, and also to help us find ways of avoiding the arousal of unwarranted guilt feelings among parents who misinterpret such findings.

4

The Mental Hygiene Role
of the Nurse in Maternal
and Child Care*

An important trend in present-day mental hygiene leads us away from the concentration of effort on early diagnosis and treatment of individuals suffering from emotional disorder, and toward the goal of identifying and altering the sets of circumstances which might lead to such a disorder. Our attention has shifted from pathology in the patient to the pathological factors in the environment.

We recognize that the most significant area of a person's environment in relation to his mental health is the complexity of emotional interrelationships which focus on him. These relationships are most significant during his early formative years, but are important throughout his life.

In any community, certain individuals have roles which make them key people for the mental health of many others. These individuals may exert a pathogenic effect on the emotional lives of others with whom they have disturbed relationships. They may be considered carriers of

*Published in *Nursing Outlook*, Volume 2, January, 1954. From a speech delivered at NLN Convention 1953.

mental ill health, similar to the carriers of typhoid and other infectious diseases.

Preventive psychiatry is attempting today to identify such key people who are disturbed and have disturbing relationships, and to ameliorate their distorted attitudes in order to prevent their pathogenic effect in the community. It is also studying the circumstances which produce such disturbed relationships in order to prevent these people from becoming mental ill health carriers. This work is being undertaken in the hope that the further back the pathogenic process can be traced, the simpler will be the factors involved and the less costly will be their treatment.

In considering the circumstances which produce disturbed relationships and also the conditions under which these have their maximum pathogenic effect, the concept of emotional crisis has become important. Whatever their prevailing emotional relationships with their fellows, people are usually in a condition of emotional equilibrium. There is some stability in their mental life whether they are emotionally ill or healthy, whether they are carriers of mental health or of ill health. Under certain conditions, however, this balance of psychic forces is upset and for a period, often quite short, the person is in a state of emotional disequilibrium. At such times of crisis, a relatively small force acting for a short time may tip the balance either to one side or to the other, and a new stable equilibrium is obtained. Such a crisis may lead a key person to develop into a carrier of emotional ill health. During the brief period of disequilibrium, a person may be more vulnerable to the pathogenic effect of a carrier. But it is precisely at such crisis periods that the mental hygienist may operate most profitably by lending his emotional strength to the healthy side of the balance of psychic forces and, with an expenditure of minimal energy, produce fundamental changes in the attitudes of people. The goal of mental hygiene, therefore, is to identify crisis periods among important people in the community, and to ensure that they will emerge from these crises with healthy interpersonal relationships so they will not become carriers of mental ill health.

Among these key people are parents, kindergarten or other teachers, army officers, foremen in industry, and similar persons whose roles place them in charge of others. Here we will discuss the mother, who has been studied more than any of the others. Although she comes into contact with a smaller number of susceptible individuals, her influence for good or ill on her young children is probably the most potent environmental factor in their emotional development.

The Influence of the Mother

In studying the circumstances which produce a disturbed mother-child relationship and turn the mother into a carrier of emotional ill health, we have learned that she goes through a period of increased susceptibility to crises which stretches from pregnancy through the lying-in period and into her child's first few years of life.

During pregnancy, the biological processes and their emotional impact stimulate the re-emergence of problems of her femininity and its association with her relationship to her own mother, which may have been only partially solved in the past. The general emotional crisis may also stir up any other personality weakness and lead to emotional disequilibrium. Problems for which solutions in the past were incomplete may be revived, giving opportunity now to find a better or a worse solution for them. Pregnancy, therefore, may lead to greater maturity and healthier relationships, or it may lead to the kind of pathogenic situation in which the expectant mother prepares to use the coming child as a partial solution for some of her problems. The danger is always present that she may relate to her child primarily on the basis of fulfilling her own need to solve these internal problems. This type of relationship, which is likely to pervert the child's development, contrasts with a healthy mother-child relationship in which the mother reacts to her child primarily on the basis of her awareness of his needs and her attempt to satisfy them.

The emotional crises of pregnancy are produced mainly through stimulation by biological processes within the mother, but after the child is born and during his early years, similar crises may be produced because the mother is stimulated from without by her intimate association with him. As he passes through successive stages of instinctual development, this association stimulates the deepest layers of her personality structure, which were laid down when she was his age. Disequilibria similar to those occurring in pregnancy, with the same range of healthy or pathogenic outcomes, may be the result.

Mental Hygiene Activities During Pregnancy and the Postpartum Period

These considerations lead mental health workers to concentrate on programs of mental hygiene supervision for the pregnant woman and the mother of young children, and the following types of activity have been among those found useful.

Ego Strengthening or General Support
This type of mental hygiene activity is nonspecific and is

likely to be of some use in most cases. Regardless of the presence or absence of crises or of their types, the worker lends his emotional support to the patient, so that her balance of psychic forces is weighted down in the direction of health and maturity. This is accomplished by the worker actively expressing an attitude of human interest and an understanding of the mother as an individual with her own characteristics and idiosyncrasies, and by accepting her as she is.

This is a very concrete and practical kind of help, but it is hard to describe. The following examples may make it clearer.

• A 31-year-old woman, after attending a sterility clinic for two years, was discharged from the clinic as a hopeless case, and she and her husband reconciled themselves with difficulty to a life of childlessness. The wife embarked on a professional career and they made elaborate plans to travel abroad in order to gain professional experience in different countries.

In the midst of these plans, the wife suddenly became pregnant and much to her own and her husband's surprise she reacted violently against it. Though she attended the prenatal clinic regularly and cooperated fully with her doctor, she was quite outspoken in her rejection of the pregnancy, and continued working until the last possible moment. She ascribed her resentment to the unexpectedness of this interruption of her carefully-laid plans, saying, "Previously when I did all I could to have a baby, I couldn't become pregnant and now when I have given it up and got going on something else, this comes along!"

The mental health workers were very interested in the underlying psychological mechanisms, but they made no active attempt to uncover them. Instead, they built up a warm relationship with the woman and encouraged her to verbalize very freely her complaints against the unpredictability of her fate. Far from urging her to accept her lot with gratitude, they made their sympathy clear to her, and let her know that they understood her negative feelings, and that they accepted and respected her just as much as they did patients who were happy with their pregnancies. This support became all the more meaningful to her as month followed weary month, and her complaints and rebellion continued unabated. She was repeatedly reassured that this free expression of her hostility to the pregnancy cast no reflection on her capacities as a potential mother, and she was supported in her hopes that when the baby would be born, her original positive attitude to motherhood would return.

Her negativism did not disappear until she went into labor. A day later when she put her son to her breast for the first time, she felt a sudden wave of motherliness sweep over her, and thereafter she behaved like all mothers who love their children.

• A 19-year-old girl had suffered since childhood from many anxieties and fears. When she became pregnant, these were intensified; in addition to her old fears of the dark, burglars, heart trouble, or dropping dead, she was terrified that her baby would die, would be born mentally defective, or be a monster, blind, or crippled.

Whenever she came to the prenatal clinic, and during frequent home visits by the nurse, she was allowed to talk freely about her fears and she was listened to with patience and sympathy. She was not reassured directly but her anxiety usually lessened when she became aware that the worker, listening carefully to her horror stories, was in no way upset by them. She was much strengthened when she found that she wasn't laughed at, or told to pull herself together, but that she was accepted as she was—a weak and nervous girl struggling hard to cope with problems that most other people hardly bother about. Any signs of strength were noted and praised and the positive feelings she had about her husband and her pregnancy were recognized and appreciated. She was surprised to find that the workers continued to respect her despite all her nervousness, which she had previously felt to be in some way morally reprehensible; and her own self-respect was increased.

She bore her labor with what was for her great bravery but almost collapsed during the lying-in period when she was faced with the responsibility of caring for her baby. She was encouraged not to breast feed and she was allowed to move very slowly in taking over the care of the child. During her first few weeks at home, the nurse made frequent visits and answered innumerable phone calls. She allowed the mother to be childishly dependent on her and accepted her very slow development toward ordinary maternal responsibility.

Little by little, this mother began to realize what she meant to her baby, who was so much more helpless than she, and whose satisfactory development soon began to bear witness to her maternal devotion. After the third or fourth month, the patient's fears lessened considerably, and with her increasing pride in her motherhood a characteristic maturing process became evident in her total personality.

It is hard in these and other cases to evaluate the importance of these techniques. A meaningful emotional relationship between the mother and an accepting non-judging worker certainly helps to strengthen the ego-integrative forces in the mother's personality. Perhaps the chief significance of such a relationship lies in its insurance value; in case of a crisis, the mother can immediately borrow strength from the worker to whom she has become attached.

Mobilizing Environmental Sources of Love and Support

The pregnant woman needs extra love just as much as she needs extra vitamins and protein. This is especially so in the last few months of pregnancy and during the nursing period. During pregnancy she often becomes introverted and passively dependent. The more she is able to accept this state, and the more love and solicitude she gets from the people around her, the more maternal she can be toward her child. Professional workers cannot give her the love she needs, but they can mobilize the members of her family, and especially her husband, to do so. In our culture, husbands and other relatives are often afraid of spoiling the expectant mother and special efforts are needed to counteract this attitude.

• A warm and sensitive young girl, married to a rather cold, intellectual, and introverted man, showed many signs of insecurity throughout pregnancy. She sometimes talked of her longing to see her mother, to whom she was much attached but who lived 30 miles away. Her husband was away at his job all day and most of the evening, so she had bought a pet dog to comfort her in her loneliness. The husband was told of his wife's increasing demands for signs of affection and said that he feared she was getting soft and childish. In a few short discussions, he was helped to ventilate his anxiety that she would become an emotional burden on him. He was then urged to spend as much time as possible at home and was reassured that her regressive passivity and increased demands for love were quite normal manifestations of pregnancy. He was advised to make special efforts to demonstrate his love as concretely as possible, both by personal attentions and by helping with the housework. He was also supported in a plan to buy a small secondhand car so that his wife could visit her mother. His relations with his mother-in-law were cool, but when he understood the importance of providing his wife with as much love and affection as possible, he readily agreed to invite his mother-in-law to stay with them during the last week of pregnancy and the first few weeks after his wife returned with the baby.

The young mother's response to these simple measures was gratifying, and she made a surprisingly smooth adjustment to the early stages of nursing and caring for her baby.

Anticipatory Guidance

This technique has been much described during recent years and will, therefore, receive only brief mention here. It is a valuable method of mobilizing the patient's strength beforehand so that she is able to meet a crisis situation more constructively. She is told in detail what to expect, and by imagining in advance what it might feel like, she is able to lower her anxiety level and to develop a readiness for a healthy reaction. It is worth stressing that the technique works best when the future events are described in greatest detail and when the patient is given a full opportunity to discuss her feelings, and particularly her anxieties, beforehand.

In order to use this method, the worker must know the usual physical and emotional changes of pregnancy, labor, and child development, and he must be able to formulate his predictions reassuringly and yet without slurring over possible sources of difficulty. Examples of topics which can usefully be discussed with every pregnant woman include the sudden unexplainable mood changes, the irritability and emotional lability, and the passivity which are so frequent in pregnancy. Possible changes in feelings about sex activity should usually be discussed as early as possible with both husband and wife. Fears and superstitions about maternal impression, difficult labor, and congenital abnormalities of various types are rendered less troublesome if these worries have been mentioned earlier by the worker as being a very significant inheritance from past ages.

Educational preparation of the expectant woman for labor has been advocated principally by the devotees of natural childbirth. It is not necessary to subscribe to this theory in order to realize the importance of this preparation. There is little doubt that a woman who has been told exactly what to expect will have a smoother and less traumatic experience in labor than someone who has no idea of what is coming next, and is therefore a prey to her imagination.

Similarly, a few short discussions ahead of time on breast feeding will pay excellent dividends, apart from helping an ambivalent woman to come to a clearer decision beforehand as to whether or not to nurse her baby. One mother felt no real love for her baby until he was three weeks old. Up to that time, she was interested in him and felt sympathetic and protective, but no more so than toward any other baby. She was not at all disturbed by this, and made a satisfactory adjustment to breast feeding because she had been explicitly warned that this lack of maternal feeling would probably occur as a temporary phenomenon. This is an extreme case, but delays of two to five days before the mother feels fully maternal are not at all unusual nor are they unnatural.

Help in Specific Crises

Intervention directed toward insuring a healthy outcome to an emotional crisis must operate at the time of the acute disequilibrium in order to achieve a maximum effect. The same effort applied after the acute phase is over will have less chance of changing the balance. For this reason it is important to learn to recognize the crises of pregnancy and the post-partum period, and, if possible, to be alert to their prodromal signs so that they can be predicted and prepared for. This is an area in which our knowledge is still very scanty, but the following examples serve to illustrate what is involved.

• A woman who had been adapting fairly well to her pregnancy suddenly became tense and anxious in her seventh month. She complained of mental confusion and ineffectiveness. She gave a history of a disturbed relationship with her mother, who had suffered a psychotic breakdown when the patient was a young girl and had been in a mental hospital for a couple of years. In the interview with the psychiatrist, the patient described with much emotion how upset she had been when her mother was taken away, and how she had had to act as mother to the rest of the family and even to her mother for years after her discharge from the hospital. In connection with her own present upset, she said that she was having a desired pregnancy and had felt fine until a week previously, when she had begun to feel passive and useless. Despite all her efforts, she could not shake off this apathy and she was now tense and sleepless. She said she was happily married but was completely frigid and had some dyspareunia.

The psychiatrist pointed out to her that her introversion and passivity were a natural reaction of her present stage of pregnancy, but that apparently she had become frightened because this sudden change in her feelings reminded her of her mother who had always been a passive and ineffectual creature. She then broke into violent weeping and said she was afraid she was going mad, like her mother. She was shown how she had made an irrational link between her passivity and her mother's illness, and she was urged to try to accept and enjoy the passivity, instead of fighting it, as a positive contribution to her pregnancy.

She was tremendously relieved and grateful for this help. During the balance of the pregnancy she was seen regularly for short interviews in which the same advice was repeated and she became relaxed. She had an easy labor and made a fairly good adjustment to breast feeding, but she required continued support during the first few months of motherhood to relieve her anxiety that she would fail as a mother. Interestingly enough, six months after the delivery she reported that she was no longer frigid and that she was planning another baby.

This girl had a deep disturbance of personality involving conflicts relating to her femininity based on traumatic experiences with her mother. Orthodox psychotherapeutic help would probably have been difficult, and certainly lengthy. When the biological changes of pregnancy precipitated her into a state of passivity, it upset her previous emotional equilibrium, in which she had defended herself against identifying with the mother's femininity by always being active and dominant. At this strategic moment, it was possible to help her to realize that passivity and femininity were not dangerous, and that she could be a woman and a mother without suffering the fate of her own mother. Offering this help—as it is possible to do in many cases—did not entail the lengthy process of giving her insight into the origin of her difficulties.

● Another woman, toward the end of her second pregnancy, began to express worries she might give birth to an ugly girl. Her first child was a girl and was very pretty. She feared that the coming baby could not be as nice and would be bound to have a hard time. She herself had been a tomboy, and her mother had favored her older sister who was pretty and feminine. Earlier in the pregnancy she had related this information with little show of emotion, but as the delivery date approached, she remembered with great vividness her childhood jealousy of her sister and her own feelings of inferiority and insecurity regarding her mother's affection. She was encouraged to talk freely about those old problems and she was shown quite directly that she was preparing to identify her new baby with herself as the younger of two girls, and was worried lest she reject it in the same way she imagined her mother had rejected her. This kind of encouragement relieved much of her anxiety but it is impossible to say how effective the intervention would have been because she gave birth to a boy.

This case is interesting as it shows the train of events leading to the use of a child to work out unsolved conflicts of the mother. It also shows how buried problems come to the surface during pregnancy, and hints at the ease with which they can sometimes be handled.

• A primipara had a smooth and normal pregnancy, but had a long and difficult labor and the baby suffered a left-sided facial paresis from forceps. The mother had a bladder injury and had to stay in bed with an indwelling catheter. For administrative reasons, the baby was cared for in a nursery on a different floor of the hospital from the mother. Because the mother was unable to see it for the first three days, she refused to believe that the baby had only a mild injury. Her tension was relieved when she was given a true picture of the diagnosis and was told that she was entitled to be depressed and was encouraged not to try to put on a bold face. She was also given supervision and supportive help during breast feeding. During this contact, she confessed that she had been blaming herself for the difficult labor and the baby's injury, feeling that she had not carried out all the instructions given her in the prenatal clinic, particularly in regard to stopping sexual intercourse at the thirty-fourth week. Her guilt in relation to this was relieved.

This is a typical example of the danger of a bad start to the mother-child relationship, and the way in which the reality of a birth injury rapidly becomes involved in the formation of guilty fantasies based on past conflicts.

● A young music student was seen in the fourth month of her pregnancy. She seemed strangely anxious about the wellbeing of the fetus and spent a long time discussing the signs of quickening. She admitted that the pregnancy had been unplanned and unwanted. A month later she was still asking for reassurance that the fetus was alive and healthy, which caused the obstetrician to suspect that she had done something to try to terminate the pregnancy. He told her that young girls who are upset at becoming pregnant sometimes try to interfere, and asked her outright whether she had attempted abortion. With much emotion, she confessed that she had done so but that she had told nobody about it—not even her husband, who was a theology student and felt that abortion was a terrible sin. She came from a religious family which also would be upset if they found out what she had done. Now she felt guilty and was sure that she had injured the baby. She felt she might have killed it, or at least if it lived to be born, it would be a monster. The obstetrician made no attempt to hide the fact that he felt she had acted improperly, but by his tone of voice and by his continued interest he made her realize that her feelings of guilt were exaggerated. Opening up the subject and giving her the chance to share her secret offered her tremendous relief; when he felt that he had lessened her guilt feelings sufficiently, he reassured her in regard to her anxieties about injuring the baby. The obstetrician's simple but timely intervention saved this girl not only from the further torture of pathological guilt and anxiety, but from a probable disorder of her relationship with the child.

We have come to recognize that a failed attempt at abortion is a potent cause of a peculiarly pathogenic disorder of the mother-child relationship. The mother typically shows great guilt in her handling of the child, feeling that she had previously attempted to murder him. She is tremendously anxious about his health, fearing that she must have injured him in some way, and by coddling and overprotection she manages to make him into a weakling whom she takes from doctor to doctor for all kinds of treatments. She feels that this sickly creature who makes such demands on her time is the punishment for her crime. Often she regards him as the visible sign of her evil and behaves cruelly to him, symbolically castigating her own sin.

Such children often appear in child guidance clinics with distorted personality structures. At this stage, it is hard to do anything for them; it is no consolation to the psychiatrist to trace the history of the disturbed mother-child relationship back to its origin in the traumatic incident of early pregnancy and to realize that a few sessions of simple treatment at that time would probably have prevented the subsequent sad development.

The Specific Role of the Nurse

Has the nurse a specialized function in this field of mental hygiene? She is a general practitioner among the many specialists who operate in maternal and child care, the obstetricians, pediatricians, nutritionists, psychiatrists, psychologists, and social workers; she must know something of each of these specialties, and yet she is not competent to operate independently in any of them. She knows this and so does the patient, which is bound to make the nurse feel insecure. The competent nurse must know the boundaries and limitations of her work. This insecurity may lead her to the defense of denying her limitations and trying to operate in the area of one of the specialists. Has she then a specialized function of her own? I feel that the answer to this question is very definitely in the affirmative.

The nurse's specialized function arises from her very special position in relation to her patient, and this is a role which is not open to any of the other specialists except under atypical conditions.

The chief characteristic of this position is closeness.

Closeness in Space
The nurse goes into the patient's home, and in the hospital she remains at her bedside. She penetrates physically into the patient's environment.

Closeness in Time
The nurse's contact with the patient can be constant and continuous. She can make home visits throughout pregnancy; she is constantly present during labor and the lying-in period and when the mother returns home she can follow her there. It is not too difficult administratively to keep the number of nurses dealing with one patient at a minimum and thus provide a unitary link right through the period under discussion. Apart from the importance of this in building up a supportive emotional relationship, its chief significance is that the nurse may often be actually present throughout a crisis situation.

Sociological Closeness
The traditional role of the nurse makes the patient regard

her as being on the same status level as herself. In the professional relationship the patient feels that the other specialists are high above her in status; she regards them as parent figures, but on this scale she considers the nurse a sibling figure. This means that communication is free and easy and involves little tension. The patient feels that the nurse speaks her language, there is no need to put on a show in front of her and she is not afraid to ask questions. In many countries this sibling role of the nurse is symbolized by the pregnant woman calling her "sister." She is traditionally not just an ordinary sister, but an especially wise one—an older sister with experience who is interested in helping.

Psychological Closeness

Linked with the sociological closeness, which is based on the patient's perception of the nurse, is the fact that the nurse maintains less psychological distance than other professionals do in treating her patients. She involves herself more freely, and uses herself more directly in a more unsophisticated and less rigid way, and with the use of fewer formalized psychological techniques. This human closeness is reciprocated by the patients, who show their feeling of freedom and ease by rapidly building up a trusting relationship.

This closeness is unique among the professional workers who are in contact with the mother and young child. The fundamental role of the wise sister, who is present in times of trouble, gives the possibility of a unique and specialized function to the nurse. It is an important heritage and must be jealously guarded, for if it is lost the specialized mental hygiene functions of the nurse will be lost with it.

Mental Hygiene Functions of the Nurse

Case Finding

The nurse has the broadest contact with the mother and her human and physical environment. She can make her observations and collect her information when the people concerned are not on their guard and putting on a show. Moreover, she is frequently present when the members of the family are together, so that she can actually observe their interactional behavior. This may throw a quicker and truer light on their interpersonal relations than hours of history taking. This allows the nurse to specialize in identifying crisis situations, and to recognize environmental circumstances which are hazardous to the interpersonal relationships of the patient and her family.

Initiation of Motivation

Having recognized a situation which is a mental health hazard, the nurse has an essential role in arousing the individual's motivation to seek the right professional help. In this work, since we are operating in a field in which symptoms often do not exist as a stimulus to seek help, and one in which the family members usually do not feel a need to involve themselves, the problem of motivation (which in the therapeutic setting is relatively simple) becomes complicated and difficult. It is a problem which in certain cases may make the biggest demands on the skills of the psychiatrist; but the nurse must make the first move because it is her link with the mother or the relative which makes the initial interview possible.

Interpretation of the Patient to the Specialists

Routing the patient to the appropriate specialist is often the nurse's function, and is managed efficiently in most clinical settings. What is usually less well managed is the interpretation of the patient and her environment to the specialist sitting in his office. The nurse moves freely between the two worlds of patient and specialist. In each she should be regarded as an equal, and it should be her function to act as an emotional and intellectual bridge between them. Too often the wealth of information she has collected about a case remains locked inside her and is not passed on to the other specialists. There are many reasons for this, but both the nurse and the other professional workers ought to try to work out a more efficient method of ensuring this essential communication.

Interpretation of the Specialists to the Patient

It is the nurse's job not only to translate the words of the specialists into the patient's language, but also to unify the prescriptions of the different specialists and help the patient accept them as part of a coherent framework. It is interesting that at the present time she has much less difficulty dealing with interpretation in this than in the reverse direction.

Emotional Support

The special way in which the nurse gives emotional support has already been stressed—she gives assistance as a "wise sister". Because of this the patient can accept her help without loss of independence or self-esteem and, therefore, usually shows less resistance. The support is available on the spot, in time of crisis, and can be of the general nonspecific type previously described.

The nurse can stimulate and build up the supportive relationship by giving advice and practical demonstrations of service to the pregnant woman for herself and the infant. Help in preparing the layette, bathing the baby, making the formula, and supervising breast feeding brings the nurse and the patient into a close collaborative relationship. These procedures should be regarded not only as opportunities for imparting knowledge, but, perhaps more importantly, as occasions for fostering and supporting the ego strength of the mother.

Teaching

Adding to the mother's store of intellectual knowledge increases her ego strength, and this is regarded as a principal mental hygiene function of the nurse. The nurse as a health educator, however, has a difficult job to perform if she wishes to avoid endangering her fundamental wise sister role. The risk is that she will adopt a teacher role in relation to her patient, and if she does so, her sociological closeness is immediately destroyed. Most people conceive of a teacher as having a higher status position than themselves; the nurse who becomes teacher becomes a parent instead of a sister.

Imparting knowledge without assuming a teacher status is a technique that has still to be worked out, but it is possible. It is important that the nurse have a systematic schedule of information to convey, but she must avoid systematic teaching sessions; she should aim at informal teaching techniques, if possible in group situations where mothers have an opportunity to teach each other. It is important to stop using the term Mothers' Classes for such groups; in leading them, the nurse should not set herself up as an expert but rather as someone who is conveying what the experts say. Above all, she should try and help the mothers clarify their own thinking and learn actively rather than receive her teaching passively.

Mobilizing the Environment

This mental hygiene function, which has been described earlier, is essentially the province of the nurse.

My contention that the nurse's closeness to her patient

is the fundamental basis for her unique mental hygiene role does not imply that I am opposed to the present efforts of nurses in this country to raise their professional status to the level of the other specialists in the field. On the contrary, I feel that the difficulties inherent in the interpretation of the patient's needs to the specialists is largely due to their perception of the nurse as a worker of lower status whose reports are not likely to be very valuable. Increasing professionalization, as a result of better preparation, would improve this situation of interdisciplinary collaboration.

In order to act as a mediator between the patient and the specialists, the nurse must be regarded by each as being at the same status level as each group. She therefore has the difficult task of being all things to all men.

The danger is that in her efforts to achieve increasing professionalization, she may strive to become a specialist just like all the other specialists; she may feel that to do so means she should give up her role of sister to her patients. I can imagine that the idea of growing from a sibling role to a parent role may be a seductive one, but I would warn against trading an immediate benefit for a long-range loss.

I would emphasize that the concept of the nurse as a wise sister involves a great challenge to nursing education. It implies a higher standard of professional education in order to merit the description "wise," and this education must be carefully planned and executed so that the nurse may retain or develop the necessary emotional qualities to allow her to be a sister to her patient. This whole problem merits the most careful consideration by those who shape the policy of the nursing profession.

Techniques of interviewing and handling patients appropriate for the nurse's use need to be studied and developed. At present, most of the techniques in this field have been developed for other disciplines and, unchanged, are not transferable without endangering the nurse's status position. There is also a need to work out how such techniques can be used without increasing the psychological distance between nurse and patient.

A technique which is immediately available for the use of nurses is that of reducing a patient's superficial guilt. An example was given in the case of the expectant woman who had failed in her attempts to terminate her pregnancy. The nurse should be taught how to identify this type of guilt, since it is a potent factor in perverting interpersonal relationships, and she should learn how to deal with the problem as a routine part of her work.

Guidelines for Future Research

The thinking of the last few years has brought us to the threshold of a great new field in mental health practice, but our basic knowledge of the details of the common emotional crises of pregnancy and infancy is still scant. We know even less about the special circumstances which are likely to produce mental health hazards. It is surprising how little scientific research has been undertaken to describe the development of the emotional life of the ordinary pregnant woman.

In order to build up mental health nursing programs which are efficient, we will have to investigate this area and determine the facts. For maximum productiveness, such research should be carried out on a collaborative team basis within a framework of all the disciplines, including nursing. This type of multidisciplinary research is difficult to organize and is very costly, but we have reached a stage where it must be regarded as essential. Examples of the situations which are likely to lead to mental health hazards and should therefore have research priority are prematurity, RH-negative mothers, illegitimacy, multiple births, failed attempts at abortion, severe illness or death of a near relative during pregnancy, birth trauma in the child, and similar situations. The aim of this research would be to develop specific categories of identifiable circumstances which lead to mental health hazards, and to provide the nurse with indications for specific action in each case.

Effects of Closeness on the Nurse

The mental hygiene work based on the nurse's closeness to her patient inevitably involves the nurse herself in emotional problems. The danger is that she will find herself in crisis situations because her own problems are stimulated by those of her patients. The closeness makes her vulnerable in this respect. The likelihood that her patients' problems may set up internal disequilibrium in the nurse is especially great in this field of maternal and child care because of its significance to every woman, and especially to a woman of childbearing age.

One unfortunate result of such a process is that the nurse might try to work out her own problems through her patients. This might show itself by the nurse usurping the mother's role and becoming possessive of the baby or being possessive of the case in relation to the other workers in the field. Another way in which the nurse might attempt to deal with her emotional upset would be by withdrawing from the possibility of involving herself with her patients, either by becoming insensitive to their problems or by increasing her psychological or sociological distance.

It must be emphasized that such emotional upsets are

likely to occur in nurses of stable personality if they are doing an efficient mental hygiene job, and must be regarded as a routine occupational hazard.

If this analysis is correct, and our experience indicates that it is, mental hygiene activity by nurses should be planned to include specific safeguards in order to protect the nurse and to minimize her working difficulties.

The best safeguard is an efficient system of technical supervision along the lines which have been worked out in casework and psychotherapy. This is a relatively new idea in nursing; proper methods and organizational framework have still to be developed.

The general nursing supervisor certainly has a part to play. By the atmosphere she creates in her unit, and by the manner in which she conducts herself in relation to the nurses, she sets the tone for their relationship with their patients. She is able to provide a background of non-specific emotional support which she expresses in her attitude of trust in the capacities of the nurses, her respect for their individuality, and her tolerance for their emotional difficulties. She can also be of limited help in some crisis situations, but her hands are bound by the demands of her leadership role which forces her to keep the relationship between the nurses and herself on a basis of strict reality. If she permits herself to become involved to any extent in their fantasies, she will usually experience difficulty in carrying out her tasks as their administrative superior within the agency's hierarchy.

For help in times of emotional crisis, the nurses need someone with whom they can have a freer emotional relationship than is possible with their supervisor—someone outside the administrative hierarchy, with whom they can share their secret emotional reactions without fear it may one day count against them on the job. This person can allow herself to be involved in their fantasy lives since she has no commitments which conflict. She can, by her permissiveness, allow the development of the special kind of relationship which can be used to help the nurses achieve a more mature solution of their problems in relation to their work.

It must be emphasized that this outside supervisor—the mental hygiene consultant—does not carry on psychotherapy with the nurses. She restricts her intervention to helping them overcome the emotional obstacles which prevent them from operating to their maximum efficiency in the case which is brought to consultation. Consultation technique aims at excluding discussion of the private life of the nurse and deals with her problems by helping her find a solution to the patient's difficulties. The benefit to the nurse is obtained vicariously when she is helped to overcome her own troubles, once removed, in her patient.

The mental hygiene consultant nurse is a new arrival, and she has hard work ahead of her in developing her techniques and establishing her position in the organizational framework of the nursing profession. That she has arrived is a welcome sign of the increasing recognition of some of the important problems outlined in this chapter.

5

The Role of the Social Worker in Preventive Psychiatry*

The following lecture is based on some ideas in preventive psychiatry with which medical social workers are probably already familiar. And, basing myself upon these newer ideas, I am going to try to think aloud about where the present day social worker may fit in.

I think perhaps the most important idea in this area is what might be called the ecological theory of emotional health. The evaluation of the state of an individual's health or ill health can be conceived of as an assessment of a type of internal equilibrium, a balance of intrapsychic forces in a more or less stable state. This is an intraper-sonal phenomenon. Significant thinking at the present time ascribes tremendous importance to the concept that what is going on inside that individual is in the present situation part of a complicated interrelated field of forces which includes not only these intrapersonal forces but also the interpersonal forces between him and the members of his relevant human environment as well as other forces in his wider social environment. The concept is that what

*Transcribed talk presented at the Annual Dinner of the American Association of Medical Social Workers San Francisco, June 2, 1955. Reprinted from *Medical Social Work*, 1955, 4 (4), 144-159.

is going on inside any individual is in dynamic interplay and is at every moment affected by what is going on outside him. If we wish to get a clear idea of what is happening, we should not divide them.

Forces Affecting the Individual

Another important point is that we are beginning to realize that for too long we have carried over into the preventive field a basic idea from the field of therapeutic medicine which is not valuable here: the concept of the individual patient as our reference point. This is a useful focus if we are dealing with an illness which is associated with structural change in an individual. We can isolate this individual with more or less relevance to our investigations and to our treatments. We focus on the patient and then we think of the forces acting upon him, the forces that acted beforehand in order to produce the pathological effect, and the forces that may act afterwards to change him either for better or for worse. When we are thinking in preventive terms, this can be a very misleading concept. We are beginning to realize that we should think of a field of forces, of a unit of the whole society—whatever size of unit—rather than of an individual patient.

Another idea which is of importance is the concept of crisis. This is associated, of course, with the idea of equilibrium, because one significant thing about a balance of forces is that it may become unbalanced. We have discovered that a state of emotional ill health in an individual is preceded at some time or another in the past by a significant period of disturbance of his previous equilibrium. The person passes through a period of emotional upset which is not in itself an emotional illness, but which leads eventually to a new state which may be the equilibrium of ill health rather than that of health. Moreover, this crisis or upset in the internal balance of forces in the individual is usually precipitated by, and is the reaction to, a disturbance in the field of forces by which he is surrounded. The outcome of this crisis, which is usually not too protracted, will determine the type of lasting equilibrium which will emerge and whether it will be a healthy or an unhealthy state.

It is very important to realize that during this period of crisis, when the balance of forces is unstable, a relatively minor force acting for a relatively short time can switch the whole balance over to one side or to the other. If we tip the balance over to one side, we switch it down to the side of an equilibrium which is one of mental health, and if we switch it down to the other side, to one of mental ill health.

During the particular period of crisis, which may be a few hours, a few days, or at most a few weeks, a small force acting for quite a short time produces lasting changes which that force could never produce beforehand or afterwards. Also, at this moment of crisis there are certain significant forces in the environment which are especially important, and of course one of the outstanding of these forces is that of the relationship of certain key people to the individual concerned. This relationship may be supportive—that is, tending to weigh the balance down in a healthy direction—or it may be weakening and destructive—and, pushing towards illness.

Even as I discuss the problem in terms of webs of relationships and how we must avoid the concept of the individual patient, I begin thinking in terms of one individual and the effect of the forces on that individual. At the same time, I realize that I have not given the whole story, and that I have to think also of the other individuals in the field. For instance, there is one experience that all of us who have worked in a child guidance clinic have had. We see a child who comes as the patient with some symptoms for treatment. We enlarge our focus and we find that he has a mother with a disturbed relationship towards him. We think that there is a causal connection. Then we do something to undo this disturbance of relationship between the mother and the child. That is fine, if we are therapeutically oriented, in which case we will say to ourselves, "Here is my patient, I must cure him." Perhaps we do cure our patient.

But many of us in the past have been rather rudely surprised to discover that if we followed up such a case and if we widened our focus just a little more, we found that maybe the father, who up to the time of therapy had been reasonably well, now becomes disturbed, or another child, or a grandparent. In other words, the more we narrow our focus, the more we do not need to take into account that our manipulations are causing change in the field as a whole. Of course, we might quite validly say we are only interested in this particular child, and yet we may find, if we are honest with ourselves and if we watch the situation afterwards, that we have benefited the child at the expense of the mother or one of the other children. And who knows (usually we are not in a position to know, because we have closed the case) whether the final reaction, even for that child, may not be worse than the first condition?

This leads me to the question of whether we can adequately analyze any emotional situation. We can. The crucial question is where do we draw the circle of our investigation? We used to draw the circle around the patient, for example, the child. At that stage all we were interested in was what was going on inside the child, in the intrapersonal difficulties of the child, and we became proficient in working out techniques of investigation and treatment for these intrapersonal difficulties.

Then we became wiser and we spread the circle of our interest a bit wider, around the mother and the child. We talked about mother-child relationships and their disturbances. And now people are getting a bit restive and are saying we ought to draw the circle a bit wider still, around the father, the mother, and the child. And when we do that, we have started on a process and begin to say we ought to take the siblings in, and maybe the grandparents. We begin to ask ourselves, "Well, now, what about the father's work situation, what influence does that have?" Then we realize that the child is not always at home; he goes to school. Should we bring the teachers in? And if we bring the teachers into our study, what about the social structure and culture? And if we are going to take that into account, what about the tensions in the surrounding community?

Eventually all these forces from outside narrow down and influence the particular child who was the original patient presented for treatment. So we can make our analyses in regard to the intrapersonal situation which the person presents, or we can add the interpersonal forces in the small group of the family. We can make a sociological analysis in regard to the structure of that particular community. We can analyze the situation anthropologically from the point of view of the systems of customs and values of that particular culture which sanction certain behavior of the individuals in that situation and give them the support and protection of the group as a whole.

The Social Worker and the Environment

It now becomes pertinent to ask ourselves where social

workers come in and what the role of the social worker is in regard to these ideas. A good way of beginning to think this out is to say that the role of the social worker will obviously be influenced and determined by her previous professional education and experience and by the kinds of skills which she has developed. It is clear from my analysis so far that she has one very obvious role, which is perhaps hardly possible to any other clinical worker, as she is the specialist in assessing environmental phenomena.

The theoretical concepts I have referred to offer the social worker new opportunities that she has not had before, and at the same time a new challenge. This concept challenges the social worker in this country to return to her vocation after a period of several years when, I feel, she has strayed from her traditional path. This she has done when she has altered her focus from the social aspects of casework to the intrapersonal aspects of psychotherapy.

I was recently talking to a visitor from Sweden who asked me whether social workers in this country make home visits. I told him that years ago social workers in the United States did a lot of home visiting. That was when they were interested in the cruder aspects of the environment. And then, as sensitive people, they became aware of certain emotional phenomena, not just of the size of the room or the arrangement of the furniture and the number of people in the family, and so on, but of the emotional factors in the environment. And that's when they came over to start a partnership with the psychiatrists. I hope I will not be considered presumptuous if I say that in developing this partnership they have been intellectually seduced by psychiatry and its philosophy of the moment.

Until recently, social workers felt that ordinary

casework had a low value. The important thing was to deal with the intrapersonal, emotional factors. This was difficult to distinguish from the kind of work which psychiatrists call psychotherapy: focusing on the intrapersonal difficulties of the client, handling him in an interview situation, and working out techniques for relieving his intrapsychic conflicts. I will not say that social workers did better or worse than the psychiatrists in terms of achieving results. If I had to train someone *ab initio* as a psychotherapist, I feel that a trained social worker would probably be a better candidate than a physician.

But the time has arrived when social workers should realize that they have, in regard to these newer concepts, a tremendous field of opportunity, which is to make use of their traditional knowledge of environmental factors, but not in the old way; they must utilize their increased knowledge of emotional factors and, most important, their knowledge of the unconscious implications of overt behavior.

The theme of the unconscious implications of overt behavior is tremendously important. It is the basis of psychotherapy, but need not be restricted to psychotherapy and to the intrapersonal phenomena. Social workers can make use of this knowledge and this sensitivity in regard to the environmental forces which impinge upon people. What, then, are these functions which the social worker might take on in regard to this tremendous field?

First, very obviously, she is the member of a clinical team who can best advise where to draw the circle in regard to the strategy of assessing a situation. This is a difficult and important question as we cannot go drawing our circle around the world. There has to be a place where the width of the circle, in terms of learning which forces are significant, has to be countered by the width of the circle in terms of being able to handle the crucial forces in a practical way. There are certain factors which are going to be critical, and certain which are not. We cannot go into history, economics, and politics; if we did, we would get nowhere. We might, in the very long run, get an accurate analysis of a particular situation; but we would not get too far from the practical point of view of doing anything about it.

A clinical team needs someone who is expert in these environmental factors to answer the questions. "Where do we draw the circle? Do we take in the school in this case? Do we take in the-local community tensions in that case? Do we take in the subcultural phenomena in the other case? Do we take in the father? The grandmother? Whom do we take into our study?"

The Social Worker and the Field

And now I come to an important practical point. In order to do this, the social worker must change her habits of work. She must go back into the field. Some start off by spending time in the field and then work their way up to having an office with a carpet on the floor. Returning to work in the field may involve the danger of loss of status, as well as being less comfortable!

The social worker can learn something about the field, no doubt, from interviewing the mother and child in his or her office, but cannot really learn the essential things she needs to know. She cannot learn what the significant parts to deal with are without actually penetrating the environment and getting the information by sensitivity to the behavior of the people therein. In other words, she will not get the implications of the factors which are operating in the field if the information is distorted by the eyes and ears, and the unconscious parataxic distortions, of someone who is himself emotionally involved in the situation. We have all discovered by now, listening to the wife's story about her husband, we are sometimes very surprised indeed when we go to meet this big, hulking brute and find a poor drippy sort of chap who would not hurt a fly. It is only by actually penetrating the field that the social worker is going to get the relevant information.

There are techniques to be worked out in regard to assessing the field situation. It is no longer the easy thing it was twenty years ago, because now we are paying attention not only to the surface manifestations but to their deeper implications. Possibly one of the reasons the social worker retired from the field into the office was because things got too complicated. Once upon a time if she went out on a home visit and someone offered her a cup of coffee, and she wanted to be polite, she took it. Nowadays she has to think, "Well, what does this mean? She offers me a cup of coffee on this visit but she didn't do this last time. What does it mean that she leaves the door of the room open? What does it mean that she suddenly raises her voice while issuing the invitation? What does it mean that 'by chance' she has neighbors visiting her? What does it mean that there's someone there in the corner she doesn't introduce me to?" These used not to be problems. These are now very complicated problems. She also has to become sensitive now to what to do. What will happen if she takes the coffee? What will it mean if she does not take it?

The Social Worker and Preventive Intervention

This problem of assessment of the relevant forces in the environment and the role of the social worker in bringing this knowledge into the clinic, is linked with another role: the social worker is able, by virtue of her skills and her education, to make a unique contribution as regards the tactical considerations in any case in working out and implementing a plan of preventive intervention. She is usually the only person who can validly say how much of the work in any particular case can be done inside the clinic walls and how much must be done out in the field, because she is the only one who really knows the field.

I would now like to turn to techniques of preventive intervention which are appropriate for the social worker. First of all, there are the techniques of direct treatment of interpersonal relationships in the narrower circle. This is an area where a certain amount of work and research has been done in recent years. As an example of such a small unit of society, let us take the family group, which we have now clearly recognized to be an intense field of forces, highly significant for the mental health of each of its members. A lowering of the general morale of this group or a disturbance of the interpersonal relationships among its members will in many instances eventually lead to emotional illness in one or another of them, and to disorders of personality development in the children.

It is interesting to note that in such situations a psychotherapist can do very little practical prevention. Why is this? Let us say that the mother's disordered relationship with her child, in a particular case, is dependent upon a disorder of her own personality—an intrapersonal disorder which manifests itself by the symptom of a disordered relationship with the child. If we are going to try to prevent the development of neurosis in the child by psychotherapy of the mother, we may succeed; but the expenditure of psychotherapeutic time will be such that our service will be indistinguishable from that of a remedial clinic. I doubt whether the Community Chest gains by paying for adult psychotherapy in place of child therapy! Nor is there any hope of community coverage.

But now we know, as has been shown in France, Denmark, Israel, and in this country, that it is often possible to repair the disorder of interpersonal relationships without becoming involved in taking on that particular person as a psychotherapeutic patient. Techniques can be worked out which will put the relationship right without the underlying personality problems having to be right at the same time. It is possible for a woman to have a healthy mother-child relationship even if she is neurotic, and it is possible for a woman to have a disturbed mother-child relationship even if her general personality is healthy. We understand this by postulating that the relationship involves only one segment of her personality. Not all her problems are going to focus on the child. Whether her personality as a whole is neurotic or not, she may attempt to solve only certain of her problems through the child.
Now we can prevent her using the child to solve her problems by means of one of these "unlinking" techniques. But then we have to ask ourselves how she is going to solve these problems. One rather good solution, from the community point of view, is that she solve her problems by developing some stable neurotic symptom. I am not putting this forward as a practical program, but let us not forget that neurosis is a community syntonic phenomenon; that is, neurosis is the individual's sacrifice for the good of the community. It is not against the community's interests until it reaches a form and a degree where it incapacitates the person to such an extent that he cannot be a reasonable, functioning member of society.

A neurotic symptom represents a solution of a conflict between the individual's interests and the interests of the community. He is solving the conflict at his own expense so that he can say, "I'm a good member of the community.

I will not be aggressive. I will not experience or gratify my instinctual desires. I will bottle them up within me."

This is important from the point of view of prevention because what we are worried about is not so much that he is going to solve his conflict on his own person, but that he may solve his problems by manipulating others in his environment, and that in this way he may affect many others. One mother with unsolved problems may distort the personality development of five or six children. One teacher or one workshop foreman who has some unsolved problems within himself may distort the personality development and the emotional equilibrium of many, many other people who depend on him. This is what we at the Harvard School of Public Health call the "carrier" of emotional disorder: the key person in a field who is important to many other people and who has the power through his relationship with them to tip them towards health or towards ill health when they are in crisis. He has disordered relationships of such a nature that he acts destructively when other people are in a crisis situation. If such a person can be detected and reached in time, it is possible to arrest this process.

This whole area has only been opened up in the last few years. The techniques which have been developed have been called by some people "child-centered treatment of the mother" or "focused casework." Other people call it "segmental treatment." Under any name, it is a technique of interview treatment of a person whereby the worker focuses and delimits the area which is going to be the content of the discussion. This means that he does not allow a free flow of nondirective material.

The worker decides what to allow into the interview and what not to let into it. The focus is kept on a narrow segment regarding the relationships of that key person with the other people—the child, or the other members of the family, or the workers in the factory. How this is done is a matter for study and research. All I wish to say here is that it can be done, and it can be done in certain cases very effectively and very quickly. I am not talking about any kind of covering up or any kind of "patting on the back" supportive treatment. I am talking about a radical operation on attitudes and relationships.

The Social Worker and Crisis

The next form of direct intervention, the techniques of which still have to be perfected by the caseworker, is direct help to an individual in crisis. In this, the social worker is operating as a direct, grassroots-level worker. She is present at the moment of crisis. She uses her specific knowledge of the gamut of successful ways of adaptation to this crisis, and her general knowledge of the way in which people relate to problems and to other people, in order to bring her emotional support into this play of forces and to tip the balance down towards a new equilibrium in a healthy direction.

This is a very pointed intervention. In order to succeed we have to know quite a lot about the crisis. We have to know quite a lot about techniques of handling people on such occasions. One important point to bear in mind is that if we press at the right time, we do not have to do it for very long and we do not have to do it very hard. At a time of crisis, when the forces at work in an individual are in turmoil, there is an opportunity which did not exist before and will not afterwards. The importance of this in regard to community planning is the opportunity for expending skilled work in the most economical way possible at the focal point.

This leads me on to the indirect techniques which social

workers may use during crisis. This idea follows from what I have just said. The social worker cannot be present herself during the crisis period of more than a fairly insignificant number of people. But we do know that there are professional workers, representatives of the community, who are normally present during crisis periods. Many of these crises—such as birth, marriage, or death—are biosocial situations. They have been recognized in a special way in every culture system. Complicated customs, habits, traditions, and folklore have been developed in connection with these periods. These appear to have been designed by the group as a whole to protect and support its individual members.

I think it is fairly certain that in a society which is fairly well integrated, where the culture is systematically sustained, there is a minimum of individual emotional breakdown. On the other hand, where a culture has become quite disorganized, as among immigrants or transplanted people who have been separated from home and who therefore, have no fixed cultural context, no stability, and no external framework or supportive scaffolding, the amount of individual emotional breakdown is significantly large.

In a stable culture there exist people who are the safeguarding, caretaking agents of the community, who are normally present at the moment of crisis in order to help individuals on behalf of the community. The biggest problem of preventive psychiatry at the present time is the question of how to help these caretaking people act in an emotionally supportive way during these periods of crisis. The word "supportive" is a rather feeble word for so very pointed a weapon against disorder at such times. The important problem is to help these caretaking people, who are on the spot at the moment of crisis, exert their pressure to tip the balance over to the side of emotional health.

Teachers and Pupils' Crises

We have done some research at the Harvard School of Public Health on this point and it is one of the main interests in the Community Mental Health program in Wellesley and in the newly established Mental Health Program in the Whittier Street Public Health Center. We call the techniques which we have been working out in order to solve this problem "mental health consultation." The mental health consultant, in this case a social worker, works with the grassroots, caretaking agents in the community with the idea of helping them handle the crises of their clients in their prime. Such caretaking agents have included nurses, teachers, kindergarten teachers, clergymen, public health officers, general physicians, pediatricians, welfare workers, and community leaders.

Early in our work we made a discovery which seemed to us to be highly significant. We found that a caretaking person such as a teacher, who did a very efficient mental hygiene job with most of her pupils, failed completely to handle the problems of a small proportion of them. We found that such a teacher with a class of thirty children would be doing a good job with twenty-five or twenty-seven of them; but in the cases in which she failed, she failed at the most important time, namely, when those particular children were passing through crisis periods. She then brought her pressure down on the wrong side of the balance from the point of view of their mental health.

When we examined these cases, we found that the type

of child with which any teacher failed, in terms of his mental health, was related to certain problems which the teacher had not been able to solve in herself. The teacher's problems, on investigation, might turn out to be primarily intrapsychic or they might very obviously be related to tensions within the school social system or between the school and the community, as in tensions between parents and the teaching staff. Whatever the facts in any individual case, it appeared to be an invariable finding that these forces eventually narrowed down onto a disturbance in the relationship between the teacher and the child at this particular time and eventually focused on the child himself. At such moments of crisis the disequilibrium of the child was usually mirrored by a disequilibrium in the teacher. In other words, not only the child, but also the teacher, both were in a state of crisis. This was usually shown by the teacher losing her professional distance from her pupil and becoming personally and emotionally involved in his situation.

The picture presented by many of these teachers when they complained about the symptoms of one of their pupils very much resembled the familiar picture of the mother complaining of symptoms in her child, which are related to a disturbance in the mother-child relationship. In the same way that such a mother, when talking about her child, can very easily be seen to be referring to her own problems, the story of the teacher in regard to her pupil's difficulties seems to have implications in regard to her own situation.

If the things said at the beginning of this lecture are remembered, such a finding should not be in any way surprising. Both teacher and pupil are reacting in a dynamic way to the web of interpersonal forces of which they are both integral components. The particular child who is complained of at any time is not chosen by chance, but by virtue of the fact that his difficulties at that moment either stimulate or mirror in some way the here-and-now problem of that teacher in the current situation in that school. There are, of course, children with some serious structural disturbance of personality which is relatively uninfluenced by the forces I am talking about. I do not refer to these, but to the much more common situation of a reactive behavior disorder in a child, which is the usual type for which teachers request advice and help. These are *disturbing* children, but usually are not particularly *disturbed* children.

When the teacher is herself in a state of crisis, she is unable to perceive the child as a separate person and is unable to be sensitive to his needs, and is, therefore, not able to help him in his trouble in any adequate way. Instead she reacts to the child's situation in terms of her own problems; since she herself has been unable to solve these, it is understandable that what she does in regard to the child is usually not very effective.

In trying to work out methods for dealing with this kind of situation there is one rather obvious fact to bear in mind. The mental health consultant cannot offer psychotherapy to the teacher. If he did so, she would probably reject it. Her private problems are her own business, and it is up to her how she wishes to handle them. She has not defined the consultation situation as one in which her own difficulties are legitimately to be discussed. The consultant, however, has been invited into that situation by the community and has been empowered by that community to interest himself in, and to protect the mental health of, that particular segment of the child population. The community, moreover, implicitly places on the consultant the responsibility to have as wide a range of vision as possible in regard to the factors influencing the child's mental health. The teacher, in so far as she is a loyal community member, accepts the consultant in this role and empowers him to take whatever action is necessary as long as it does not explicitly impinge upon her own personal rights. It is in this framework that the technique which we have called "mental health consultation" has been evolved.

Mental Health Consultation

I can describe this technique only briefly here. A preliminary paper has appeared on this subject in the January, 1954, issue of the *American Journal of Orthopsychiatry*. This is a paper I wrote jointly with Jona Rosenfeld, a social worker from Israel, on mental health consultation in an organization for immigrant children, in which we described techniques we had worked out for helping the staff of the residential institutions deal with their problems in regard to handling the children. The technique consists of the consultant entering the child's environment and building up a relationship with the caretaking person, whom we call the consultee. Through the medium of this relationship, he gathers information on two levels. First, on the explicit level, the consultant gets a good deal of information about the details of the disturbance in this particular child, factors and forces of the disturbance in this particular child, and the factors and forces impinging upon him from the environment. At the same time that this explicit information is being gathered, the consultant is constantly sensitive to the subsurface implications of the details and manner in which the story is told in regard to the crisis situation of the consultee and of the consultee institution.

These facts can only be picked up by implication and by reading between the lines because the consultee probably regards this situation as a professional one into which she should not explicitly intrude her private problems. But since these problems are pressing upon her and since at the moment she is emotionally upset, she cannot help communicating something about them in a nonverbal way. She thinks she is talking about the child. She is, however, in everything she does both in regard to the child and in her relationship with the consultant, talking about the things that are going on inside her. As long as this is only by implication and is not made explicit, she feels the situation to be quite safe. One essential point in the mental health consultation technique is that the consultant does not interfere with this defense structure of the consultee, and never makes explicit the direct link between the problems of the child and the problems of the caretaking person. Should he do this, he immediately becomes involved in a psychotherapeutic situation which is always associated with problems of dealing with resistance. Such problems cannot be dealt with in the fluid situation of a consultation relationship.

The consultant has to pick up the implicit message which is being communicated without interfering with its nonverbal character. He must also learn to reply to this message in a similar nonverbal way, and his implicit communication must be designed in such a way as to support the emotional strength of the consultee and help tip her balance of forces towards a healthy equilibrium. In this communication the consultant must accept the defenses of the consultee and must not interpret or uncover in an explicit way things which the consultee does not wish to face at the moment.

The consultee does not say, for example, "I have unsolved problems in my relationship with my mother which are at the moment being stimulated because the headmistress of the school is a motherly person and I am at the moment in conflict with her." This is too difficult a problem for her to talk about with a comparative stranger, and it may even be so difficult that she is unwilling to think clearly about it herself. Instead, she brings up a child for discussion with the consultant and she draws particular attention to the fact that this child is, at the moment, in conflict with his mother. This is very likely not an artificial construction; the child may very well be having troubles with his mother.

But if all the consultant recognizes is that aspect, he is missing the main point of the consultation, which is why this consultee brings this child in at this moment. A few months later this teacher would probably ask for help with some other child presenting some other problem, and might not feel at all disturbed about the first child. The reason that she asked help for this child at this moment is that at this moment this particular problem is important to her. She is disturbed by it; she is in crisis over it.

The way in which such a situation is handled, in this technique, is that the consultant discusses the problem by keeping it centered around the details of the child's difficulties. He discusses the child with a constant awareness of the implications of what he is saying in regard to the consultee's problems. This results in a sort of three-cornered situation, where the consultee and the consultant are discussing the consultee's difficulties under the guise of talking about the child. One of the things which makes this technique so difficult is that the content in regard to the child must be meaningful at that level, and the consultant must constantly be killing two birds with one stone.

I hope that we soon will have worked this new technique out sufficiently to be able to present it in a systematic way to other workers. It is complicated, but it is a fascinating technique and certainly it is, potentially, tremendously important in this field. If it does not turn out to be what we want, then we must find something else that will do the same job. We must work out methods whereby a small number of highly trained people can work with the many caretaking agents of a community who are in so strategic a position during crisis periods to affect the mental health of so large a proportion of the community. If we can succeed in working out some technique of this nature and if we can get ourselves trained in it, we will have developed for the very first time a potent instrument whereby we may achieve some kind of approximation of community coverage.

The Social Worker and the Clinic Team

I do not need to say very much about the social worker's responsibilities to the clinic team, but I wish to underline two aspects of the social worker's role. First, I believe that it is the job of the social worker, by virtue of her background and her long and arduous training in dealing with her own emotions in the professional setting, to spread among the other team members a willingness to admit and accept emotional disequilibrium not only in the patients and clients but also among the staff members themselves. Some of us do not realize how very difficult this is for the other people in allied professions to understand because we may have already forgotten how long a time it took us to learn it ourselves, and to learn a tolerance of our own humanity.

The second important contribution of the social worker to the team depends upon her knowledge of the supervisory process and of the importance of emotional support for the individual worker at moments of stress. By virtue of this knowledge, the social worker can help the team build up an atmosphere which will be supportive of its individual members, so that when they go out into the field where they will be exposed to all kinds of emotional stresses, they will go out not as individuals, but as emissaries of the group. Teachers in schools of social work must be very familiar with this problem. I believe that social workers have discussed it and dealt with it more effectively than psychiatrists, and by now must have amassed a considerable body of knowledge which might be made available.

These are among the most valuable contributions which a social worker may make in a clinical team. The social workers and I have managed to make some reasonable contribution along these lines in our Family Health Clinic at Harvard. We did not manage this entirely without difficulty both for ourselves and for our colleagues. People may after all be very competent in their practice of the allied professions without having learned how to be comfortable about their own personal emotional involvement in a professional problem. It was not surprising that some of our colleagues were, in the beginning, rather ashamed to say, "Oh, I hate this patient. She really gets in my hair." Nowadays they are beginning to be able to say such things and to feel confident that they will not be rejected by the other people on the team, but on the contrary, supported in their efforts to disentangle their own emotional upset from the presenting professional problem. It is a source of great relief to an individual team member to know that the group will help him to avoid transferring onto his relationship with his client his own disequilibrium of the moment.

This certainly does not mean that I am suggesting that the social worker treat the problems of her fellow team members psychotherapeutically. It does, however, mean that she says to them, in effect, "You are entitled to have your emotional problems, and I have them too. We all have them, but they need not necessarily interfere with our work. As long as we stand together, we can have our personal problems and still do a good job. In any case, we cannot and need not deny that we, too, have emotions which may be disturbed, since this is after all one of the essential attributes of our common humanity."

Implicit in all I have tried to say is that the consideration of this topic of the role of the social worker in preventive psychiatry, at present, throws up many questions and very few definite answers; but some of the questions and some of the attempts at answers point to fascinating and challenging new vistas. For the first time we have glimpses of attainable, practical goals, but it is clearer than ever before that much hard research lies ahead. In this exciting work the social worker has an honorable and difficult part.

6

Practical Steps for the Family Physician in the Prevention of Emotional Disorder*

The etiology of emotional disorder in any individual case is very complicated. Many interacting factors are involved, including those based on constitution, childhood experiences, later life problems and their solution, and details of the unfolding of the processes of growth and development in interaction with the forces of the emotional and material environment.

If one looks at this problem from an epidemiologic point of view it is still complicated, but it is simpler: by this I mean a study of the factors in one community which are responsible for its having a higher incidence of cases of emotional disorder than another community. Such studies isolate certain common factors which operate to influence all members of a community. These factors do not determine the fate in any individual case, but they lead to communitywide differences in the frequency of certain psychological illnesses.

Viewed from this standpoint it is possible to discover certain general factors which can be combated on a com-

*Reprinted From The Journal of The American Medical Association, July 25, 1959, Vol. 170, pp. 1497-1506. Copyright, 1959, by American Medical Association. Based on a lecture read before the Honolulu Medical Society, August, 1957.

munitywide level. Programs to alter these factors may not affect the fate of any particular person but are likely to reduce the number of cases which occur during a subsequent period in that community.

In connection with these factors the following consideration seems important: The mental health of an individual is dependent on the continuous satisfaction of special requisites in the patterns of his psychological interaction with certain other people. We can speak loosely about a person having psychological needs which have to be satisfied in his interactions with others. The most obvious need is the basic psychological stimulation of having people to talk to. For years we have realized that isolation has a potent harmful effect on mental health. For centuries men have tortured their fellows by marooning them on desert islands, by solitary confinement in prisons, or by ostracism in the social setting. The list of needs also includes the opportunity to give and receive love and affection, to be dependent and to be depended on, to satisfy cravings to be controlled and to control, and to be a member of a social group in which one's identity and personality are respected and accepted, so that one's achievements are rewarded by praise and one's difficulties are lightened by sympathy and understanding.

In all cultures there exist within the structure of the society small groups of people who are bound together by significant emotional ties, and within these groups the psychological needs of the individual members are satisfied. Biological ties are usually the basis of these fundamental groupings, and some form of family structure is universal. In different cultures the pattern of families varies, but, whether one studies the small family of modern Western urban culture, the large extended family of earlier Western rural culture, or certain present-day Oriental cultures, or the matriarchal families of other cultures, we find that certain roles or tasks of psychological significance are alloted by tradition to each of the family members, that the sum of these tasks usually satisfies the needs of all the members, and that this sum is distributed among the members of the group so that no necessary role is left out.

In recent years we have discovered that the interactive possibilities afforded by the intact structure of the family are as necessary to mental health as the provision of adequate nutritional supplies are to physical health. When the traditional pattern of any family is altered by situational factors, the mental health of its members is endangered. This danger is greatest for the younger children, in the same way that nutritional deficiencies are most dangerous during early developmental phases, but the danger is also present for the mature adults.

Another similarity to physical nutrition is that if all goes well we do not usually realize the importance of these factors. The satisfaction of needs in an intact family takes place silently and automatically. It is only when the family structure is deficient that difficulties become obvious; since families are ubiquitous it has taken us a long time to realize the obvious fact of their importance for mental health and the close connection between defects in their structure and subsequent emotional disorders among certain of their members.

Importance of the Family Physician in Promoting Mental Health

From all this it follows that professional workers who deal with people as members of a family have a special place in programs of mental health promotion. The family physician is a worker with a uniquely important role in this regard. He is usually called in to a family to handle symptoms of physical disorder in one or more of its members. In dealing with this traditional task he may well add another dimension to his practice and focus his interest on those elements of the situation which involve dangers to the social structure of the family group, therefore involving dangers to the future mental health of its members. The concept of the family as a unit, and the physician as a worker with responsibilities to the whole unit, implies not only that he may accept as a patient any individual family member but also that when he is called in to deal with the symptoms of one member he will widen the focus of his interest to include all the others, whether from the point of view of their involvement in the etiology of his patient's condition or from the point of view of the effects of his patient on them as a group. This responsibility has been clear for years in cases of contagious disease, but we now realize that it applies equally, if not more so, to the social and psychological side-effects and sequelae of any illness. This latest insight is, as is often the case in medicine, a reformulation of old traditional knowledge; the family physicians in our parents' generation understood this quite well, although they may not have been able to spell it out as explicitly as we can nowadays. Increasing complexity in the medical sciences, increasing specialization, and increasing concentration on the exciting new discoveries in somatic medicine have to some extent pushed these old insights into the back of our minds. In the hurly-burly of busy practices, and in the absence of strong protagonists, they have fallen into disuse.

Moreover, the older training of physicians by the apprentice system allowed young men to acquire many of the skills of psychosocial management of the family by modeling themselves on the practice of experienced preceptors. The knowledge they acquired was not to be found in books but in the life situations of their apprenticeship. Nowadays the old type of apprenticeship is usually missing, and the books still say very little about all this—at least very little that is useful at a practical level—because the writers of these books have usually not carried out their studies within the framework of the actual situations of general medical practice but in the very specialized and unique conditions of psychiatric clinics and psychological laboratories.

Exhortations by psychiatrists that the family physician should play his part in promoting mental health are no great help. The family physician asks, "Exactly how should I do this?" and the psychiatrist usually has no concrete answer. In this chapter I will attempt to begin to give a concrete answer—or at least to indicate specific avenues for practical exploration.

Before ending this introduction, I would like to mention one other point which supports the importance of the family physician in community programs of preventive psychiatry. He is one of the key community workers who has contact with people when they are in a state of crisis. Physical illness may be a turning point which determines a change in the whole course of a person's existence; it is important to realize that during the relatively short period of the few weeks or months of the illness all kinds of decisions may be made and all kinds of psychological reorientations, as well as alterations in the structure and functioning of families, may be worked out which will affect the type of interpersonal relationships and character of intrapersonal functioning for a long time to come.

Psychiatrists have recently joined the ranks of those who are very interested in the way people solve the emotional and social problems of periods of life crisis. Previously, it was mainly novelists and dramatists who were interested in this topic, but nowadays we psychiatrists realize that the future mental health of people may be determined at crisis times by the quality of their problem-solving methods. One type of solution of a set of problems may lead to greater mental health, which explains why many people become more mature as a result of satisfactorily overcoming life's difficulties. Another type of solution may lead to mental ill health, either immediately or in the future, and either directly for that individual or indirectly for his dependents due to damage of his emotional relationships with them.

People become emotionally disturbed during these crisis periods, but the anxiety, depression, tension, and hostility are not to be confused with symptoms of psychiatric illness, which they superficially resemble. They are the signs in the emotional sphere which show that an active struggle is in process inside that individual in his attempts to wrestle with his problems. At the end of the few weeks of crisis these symptoms will disappear, once some kind of solution has been achieved. This solution may be a healthy one. On the other hand it may be an unhealthy one, and in that case either at once or in the future the individual will manifest neurotic or psychotic symptoms which represent a pathological way of dealing with his life problems through some form of irrational and psychologically distorted pseudo-solution.

The most important point for preventive psychiatry is that the type of problem solving during a crisis can be powerfully influenced by the helpful or hindering intervention of other people, both in the family circle and from the outside, in the form of the physician and other community agents. When the balance of forces is upset in a crisis a minimal intervention may produce major and stable results by determining to which side the balance will come down.

This means that the operations of the family physician during any of his visits for whatever reason to a family in crisis may have a major effect on the pattern of resolution of that crisis and on the members' future mental health.

I wish now to concentrate on examples of certain practical implications for the operations of the family physician that arise out of these theoretical considerations.

Safeguarding the Integrity of Family Structure

The general practitioner has many opportunities in his practice to help keep families from breaking up temporarily or permanently; or, if this can not be avoided, to help them find substitutes for roles which the family break-up has left vacant.

Most important is the prevention of separation of the mother from the family circle or from one of her children. Bowlby and other workers have shown fairly conclusively that the separation, for any appreciable time, of the stable mother figure from a child during the first few years of its life exerts a damaging effect on the development of the child's personality, leading in severe cases to extreme forms of psychological and psychosomatic illness. If the physician is aware of this, he will be alert to explore practical alternatives to any plan for removing a mother or a child from the home because of illness. Often the removal from home is inevitable because the nature of the illness demands hospitalization, but frequently the physician may be able to plan for this absence to be short and for the remainder of the treatment to be carried out at home. The fact that the mother is physically incapacitated certainly will influence her ability to fulfill many of the demands of the mother role, but her mere presence in the home will allow her, through repeated contacts with other family members, to maintain the emotional bonds of comfort and sympathy and mother love which are the emotional nutrients the others need.

Of course such a plan implies the need for nursing and homemaker services to care for the patient at home and to take over her housewifely duties. The physician should be active in helping the family secure such services either from the ranks of the extended family of grandparents, aunts, sisters, and cousins; from neighbors and friends; or, if these are not available, from professional workers. When the latter are not available I believe that local physicians should actively campaign among appropriate community agencies for their provision. Family physicians should be as interested in the adequacy of community agency provision in this area of homemaker services as they are in the standards of their local hospitals, since both affect the quality of the professional care they can give their patients.

The feeling in regard to hospitalization of young children should be that of avoiding or postponing or shortening it whenever possible. With modern methods of diagnosis and treatment and effective home nursing, many types of cases which in the past necessitated admission to children's hospitals can be treated at home.

When separation is inevitable the physician should encourage frequent and regular visiting to maintain channels of communication and continuation of the emotional links.

In 1952 in England, as a result of Bowlby's researches, the Ministry of Health issued a directive to permit and encourage daily visiting in children's wards. In the United States this is also becoming common pediatric practice, and some new children's hospitals have facilities for parents to sleep in the ward near their child and help with certain nursing procedures. This has led to inevitable complications in ward management and new problems for the nursing staff, but none of these have proved insoluble and they are a small price to pay for the results in terms of the safeguarding of the personality development of the children.

The physician interested in the whole family should also be on the alert for the neglect of the other children when one child is hospitalized. He should try to mobilize the efforts of other family members to cover the hiatus left when a mother is concentrating her efforts on the ill child, and his activity in this regard should not stop when the ill child comes home. We are familiar with many cases of neurotic disturbance in children which started during periods of parental neglect due to the illness of a sibling.

If the mother has to go into the hospital, the physician should try to promote communication from her to the other family members, particularly the children, through frequent verbal and written personal messages; he should also use his best efforts to help the rest of the family stay together in their home. If the family stays together they may close their ranks and take over, as a group, some of the absent member's functions, whereas if they are split up this group strength is dissipated.

In order to keep the family together the physician may have to mobilize other family members to come in and do the housekeeping, or he may have to call in a homemaker. Placing the children as individuals in other homes may seem the easier way, but it is actually more expensive in both the short run and the long run.

Another area where the family doctor can give invaluable mental health help is that of helping the father take over some of the maternal role left vacant by the absence of his wife. Husbands may need support and explicit encouragement and advice in mothering their children during this period and in assuming unaccustomed leadership in housekeeping. Some men may be rather inhibited in doing what is needed because of false feelings of shame about such activities being effeminate. The physician can watch out for this and throw the power of his prestige behind the medical prescriptions to the hesitant father.

When the separation of the mother is permanent due to death or desertion, the physician should interest himself actively in helping the family plan for her replacement by a substitute. Assistance in this direction, as in the other issues which have been mentioned, may be obtained from a family social agency; but the family physician, who is the professional person with continuing contact and responsibility for the whole family, should help in mobilizing this assistance and should coordinate these activities with his own and with those of other helping agents such as clergymen and teachers.

The physician should be equally active if it is the father and not the mother who is separated from the family by illness, death, or social factors, such as employment demands or wartime needs. A wife needs her husband's support, and children need the controlling influence of a father figure. This issue has been relatively neglected until recently. Interest in it has now been aroused by the realization that many common disorders of personality development in children, which lead to delinquency, have been influenced by the absence of a stable controlling father during the child's upbringing, so that the external discipline which is the precursor of the internal discipline of the socialized person has been missing or defective.

If there is no man in the house, the role of discipliner of the children devolves largely on the mother, and she may need the support of the physician, himself a potent *father* figure, in order to add this to her other roles. It may also be possible for him to help her out directly in certain crisis situations and to invoke the help of teachers and recreational group leaders.

Perhaps by now it seems that I am advocating turning the general practitioner into a social worker. Nothing is further from my intention. His primary role must remain that of the practitioner of the healing arts; but if our talk of treating the whole person rather than the diseased organ is to be more than a mere slogan, we must expect the physician to add an interest in some of the above psycho-social points to his traditional preoccupation with physicial functioning. The family physician may well realize that his role in the family provides him with both the responsibility ·and the opportunity to affect its functioning in ways which will have direct effects on the health of its members. So long as mental health and mental illness were conceived of as being quite separate from physical health and physical illness, the physician could afford to neglect some of these issues; but nowadays such a dichotomy is hard for most of us to accept and very hard indeed for the general practitioner who deals not with bits of people or special aspects of their functioning, as isolated in special clinics, but with the whole fabric of life within the family circle in the home.

Safeguarding Healthy Relationships

The satisfaction of individual psychological needs in the family is dependent not only on the preservation of the integrity of its structure but also on the quality of the enduring interpersonal relationships among its members. The mother may not be geographically separated from her child, for example, but her prevailing feelings toward him may be so anxious, ambivalent, or rejecting that she cannot perceive his needs, or, if she does, she may have no interest in satisfying them.

Once disordered relationships between family members have fully developed, treatment by a psychiatric specialist is usually needed to improve them; unless such intervention is forthcoming, a significant proportion of the people will eventually need psychotherapy for manifest psychiatric illness. In the past few years, however, we have discovered that the disordered relationships which are harmful take quite a time to develop to their full pathogenic intensity and that during this period the family physician may interrupt this harmful development. His helpful intervention can best be focused at certain crucial periods when disorders in relationships are most apt to occur in response to characteristic temporary situational factors.

Pregnancy

One such crucial period, both for the development of the mother-child relationship and for the other interpersonal relationships in the family, is the period of pregnancy. The mother's relationship with her new baby does not begin at his birth but is being built up during her pregnancy; the complicated metabolic development of this period has a characteristic effect on her emotional functioning, which in turn has reverberations on the emotional life of the family as a whole. These reverberations may lead to changes in the way the family members relate to the expectant mother and to each other, and these changes may become stable and may have far-reaching consequences for mental health by altering the pattern of need satisfaction within the family circle.

Recent studies on the emotional manifestations of normal pregnancy have yielded information about characteristic series of emotional changes which occur in many expectant mothers and which are apt to frighten them and to interfere with family life. The physician who knows the details of this predictable development may make powerful use of this knowledge.

His main technique will be anticipatory guidance, whereby he warns the patient and her husband ahead of time what to expect and thus gives them the chance of preparing themselves psychologically for the difficulties. For instance, quite early in pregnancy the physician should have a joint interview with husband and wife and let them both know that many women become more irritable and more sensitive than usual during pregnancy because of complicated and little-understood somatopsychic factors; therefore, if in this case the expectant mother suddenly gets angry with minor provocation, laughs or weeps for no adequate reason, or has sudden attacks of depression, neither she nor her husband need get alarmed. These changes, however dramatic, are not preliminary signs of psychiatric illness and they will disappear after delivery.

At this early conference the physician will also be well advised to mention the likelihood of changes in the pregnant woman's sexual desire and performance. Changes in appetite are frequent in pregnancy, and this relates not only to foods but to sex. In regard to this topic the physician not only gives needed anticipatory guidance but often is able to act as a channel of communication between husband and wife in relation to topics which in our culture may not be easily discussed between them. In the absence of necessary knowledge and in the presence of communication blocks so that difficulties cannot be worked out by discussion, tensions may easily arise between husband and wife based on distorted interpretations of each other's attitudes. A wife, not infrequently, gets very upset if she loses her sexual desire or capacity for orgasm; she imagines she has become permanently frigid or that she is losing her love for her husband and that he will reciprocate in kind. A husband sometimes fears that his wife is rejecting him because he made her pregnant, and sometimes he seeks alternative sources of sexual satisfaction as a reaction to this imagined rejection. Such unfortunate fantasies can be easily alleviated by the physician's prior discussion of the realities of the situation. He can also help both parties become aware of the strain under which each will be laboring during pregnancy and help them pay special attention to the need to support and sympathize with the partner's difficulties and to make allowances for signs of tension.

Such joint interviews with husband and wife, which should if possible be repeated at least once or twice more during the pregnancy, have a more essential function than just the smoothing out of expected difficulties in the marital relationship, important as this is. My studies have shown that toward the middle of pregnancy most women become more passive and demanding of affection than usual. Instead of being the giving person in the home, actively attending to the needs of others, they now turn in on themselves and feel the need to sit around and be waited on. My studies have also shown that the adequate satisfaction of these needs for increased attention and affection is not only important for increasing the expectant mother's comfort but also plays an important part in preparing her for adequate motherhood in the first few months after delivery. If she receives enough affection during pregnancy, she can give out enough affection to the baby. Those women who are deprived during pregnancy later have a tendency to deprive their babies.

Recognition of this by the physician allows him to play an important role in ensuring adequate emotional supplies at the crucial early period of the newborn infant's life. He cannot give the expectant mother affection himself, but he can try to make sure she gets it from the natural sources. There are many cultural and psychological factors which may block a husband's demonstrations of affection during pregnancy. He may be so irritated by his wife's petulant behavior and by her inability to afford him his usual sexual satisfaction that he turns away from her. He may be frightened by her increased demands, and he may feel she is changing her personality and becoming lazy and spoiled. He may resent what he feels is her exploitation of the privileges of pregnancy. His feelings of security in his manly role, which are in our culture often weakened by the lack of respect we pay to expectant fathers, may be further endangered by his wife's demands that he take over some of her maternal functions in the work in the house or caring for the other children.

The physician has the opportunity during his joint conferences with husband and wife, or if necessary during an individual interview with the husband, to prevent the difficulties which may emerge from these factors. He can reassure the husband as to the normality of his wife's reactions and as to their temporary nature, and he can enlist the husband's active help in preparing for the baby by, as it were, "charging up his wife's battery of affection," so that she can eventually pass the emotional supplies on to the baby. Most important, the physician can by his own attitudes during these meetings help increase the husband's feeling of respect for the importance of his own role as an expectant father. This may help to prevent a not infrequent cause of family difficulty after the baby arrives, when some fathers are hampered in their paternal role by feelings of jealousy in regard to the baby.

I do not wish to leave this very brief reference to the physician's preventive role in emotional disorders originating during pregnancy without mentioning the results of some recent research which has specific practical implications. My studies have shown that certain traumatic events occurring during the period of pregnancy exert a powerful harmful effect on the future mother-child relationship. Such events include the severe illness or death of a near relative of the expectant mother, particularly of a parent, her husband, or one of her children. It is very easy for the woman to displace some of her painful feelings about such an event onto her relationship with her unborn child, and her attitudes toward him get distorted by irrational ideas, such as identifying him as a reborn representative of the dead person or blaming him and sacrificing him because of unresolved feelings of personal guilt in connection with the bereavement. The physician should be especially on guard to ensure an adequate process of mourning along lines I will describe below, and he should help the mother to see and to feel that her new baby is an individual in his own right and has to be recognized and treated as a person with quite a separate fate from everyone else, including the dead person.

Abortion

Another traumatic event during pregnancy which is likely to have a major harmful effect on the future mother-child relationship is an attempt by the mother to abort herself, if this act is against the rules of her culture and traditions, and especially if she keeps it as a guilty secret. It is this guilt which blossoms in secret fantasies and which invades and distorts the relationship with the child. If nothing is done about it, the chances are high that a particularly pernicious disorder of the child's personality will eventually be produced. The important point is that this pathological sequence of events can usually be easily interrupted by the family physician, if he identifies either during pregnancy or soon afterward what has happened. The technique to be used is one which is not usually a part of the general practitioner's therapeutic armamentarium but one which can be fairly easily learned, namely, specific reduction of conscious guilt. I have discussed this at some length in a recent paper, and here I will only mention it briefly. It consists essentially of the physician helping the woman to talk about what she has done in two to three short interviews, in which he adopts an understanding and nonjudgmental attitude toward her behavior, without in any way pretending that what she did was a good thing and yet with the clear demonstration that despite what she has done he continues to accept her as a worthwhile person.

Direct Help to People in Crisis

The traditional role of the physician brings him into contact with many people during the critical period when they are wrestling with acute life problems, and at such times he can exert a particularly powerful effect on their mental health by steering them toward adequate solutions and away from maladaptive solutions. The clearest example of this is in connection with problems of bereavement.

Bereavement
Eric Lindemann, my colleague at Harvard, has carried out some interesting studies on the nature of the process of mourning which carry clear and specific implications for medical practice. He has found that a bereaved person goes through a well-defined process in adapting to the death of the relative, that this process usually takes four to six weeks to complete, and that it is characterized by a succession of specific psychological steps with accom-

panying emotional side effects. It seems that when a key figure is removed by death or desertion from a person's life, that person has to work quite hard, psychologically, in order to adapt to the loss and in order to fill in the resulting emotional hiatus.

Lindemann also found that whereas the majority of people manifest these characteristic mourning reactions, which show they are satisfactorily doing their "grief work," and recover their psychological and psychosomatic equilibrium by the end of the four to six weeks, a small but significant group of bereaved people do not show these changes, or show them in distorted form; many of these people either immediately or later show definite and sometimes extreme signs of psychiatric or psychosomatic illness, particularly depression and disorders of the gastrointestinal tract, such as peptic ulcer or ulcerative colitis.

Lindemann postulates a direct causative link between the absence of a normal mourning process and the later development of these illnesses. He has also shown that sometimes these illnesses can be interrupted by helping the patients revive the problems of their bereavement and belatedly do their undone grief work.

Among the characteristic manifestations of a healthy mourning reaction are withdrawal of interest from the affairs of daily life and business, feelings of mental pain and loneliness, weeping, disorders of respiratory rhythm with frequently repeated deep sighs, insomnia, loss of appetite, and——most characteristic—preoccupation with the image of the deceased person, usually in connection with the revival of numerous memories of joint activities with him. Lindemann feels that this last phenomenon is the key to understanding the essence of the mourning process. The bereaved person withdraws his energy from most of the aspects of everyday life and concentrates it on reviewing, detail by detail, those aspects of his past life which were enriched by his association with the deceased. In each of these life segments he has to realize afresh the pain of his loss and rather concretely to experience its permanence. In each of these segments he has to make a special act of resignation to the inevitable. This can only be achieved through suffering, but not until it is completed can the person achieve mastery and independence in that segment of his life, so that he can return to normal activity and emotional stability.

Each bereaved person must do this grief work for himself, and mourning is a lonely process; but the traditions of most cultures illustrate to us that neighbors and friends and representatives of the larger community can help the mourner both by the general emotional support of condolence and by practices which permit him or encourage him to go through the steps of his grief work. In our modern culture the weakening of religious and other cultural systems of values and traditions has thrown many people largely on their own emotional resources, and the family physician is one of the people whose work may call him to step into the breach. In doing so in this area he may well try to enlist the support of the priest or clergyman or rabbi, each of whom has his own traditional approach to these problems.

In order to understand specifically what the family physician might do to help the bereaved person mourn successfully, it is helpful to list some of Lindemann's findings among the unsuccessful mourners, who later developed various illnesses. No single simple picture was characteristic of this group, but combinations of the following reactions were common. Instead of withdrawing interest from daily life many of them showed more business activity than usual and by diverting their interest to the problems of outside life appeared to escape the inner turmoil of mourning. They did not weep. They felt little or no pain, either saying they felt numb and empty or showing a strange cheerfulness. Many of them showed marked hostility, often directed toward the physicians and nurses who had cared for the deceased. In all cases there was an absence of preoccupation with the deceased, and on direct questioning many said they were quite incapable of recalling in memory the image of the deceased person. The over-all picture which was most commonly found was an attempt to deny the emotional importance of the whole business and to get on with problems of living without the burden of mourning. In the short run the external emotional manifestations of this group seemed easier and happier than the group of active mourners, but in the long run many of them paid very dearly for their temporary ease.

The guideline for the physician who wishes to profit from these studies is to try and help his patients grieve along the lines of the first group and to be particularly active in giving his help whenever he recognizes in one of his patients, during the mourning period, signs which resemble those of the maladaptive group. Experience has shown that to help such people grieve successfully it is not necessary to know the inner psychological reasons for their being hampered in this regard. The uncovering of these deeper complications is not necessary; all that seems important is to get them by whatever means to dwell on the image of the deceased and to go over and over in their minds the many activities which they shared with him in the past, in order little by little to realize that from now on he will be missing from their lives. What is also necessary is for the physician to give the patient the full measure of his emotional support and sympathy in bearing the pain of this process and for him to mobilize other sources of support within the family and outside it. In this regard the physician should realize that emotional support depends, among other factors, on the quantity of personal interaction, so he should realize the special importance of even short extra visits to his patient during the mourning period, or, if these are not possible under the pressures of a busy practice, at least of phone communication. Since the pathological sequelae of inadequate mourning are usually so severe, these extra visits are well worthwhile.

When the physician is not able on his own to stimulate a proper mourning reaction, when his efforts to enlist the aid of ministers of religion and members of the extended family also lead nowhere, and when mourning is absent or continues without apparent resolution long after the expected period of four to six weeks, the physician would be well advised to take active steps to refer the patient to a psychiatrist at that stage and not wait for the psychiatric illness to develop. This is a situation where a specialized "stitch in time" may well "save nine."

Other Crises

Space does not permit me to go into detail about other examples of direct help by the physician to people in crisis, and I hope that some general principles may have emerged from my discussion of help with bereavement. I wish, however, to make brief supplementary mention of two other crises commonly met in medical practice, the crisis faced by parents who have to adapt to the realization that their baby has a congenital abnormality or is mentally defective and the crisis of a patient or his relatives having to adapt to a chronic or an incurable illness, a major disability, or to death itself. These situations all call for special activity on the part of the physician, in addition to the customary "frank" or "not so frank" talk.

The physician must face the fact that the impact of the

news of the diagnosis is likely to be followed by a period of psychological reorientation similar to the grief work of the mourning period and interestingly enough also lasting for about four to six weeks. Patients and their relatives should not be expected to handle these psychological burdens on their own. They may need a good deal of support from the physician in facing the painful implications of the situation and help in avoiding facile escape into denial or obliteration of the problem by wish-fulfilling fantasies. The physician should try to help them keep the problem in consciousness during this period and deal with its implications piece by piece. It is remarkable the power that ordinary people have to adapt to reality, however unpleasant. It is not realities but dreams which "make cowards of us all," and insofar as the problem is allowed to sink into dreams and into fantasies it gets removed from the strength which derives naturally from our universal adaptive mechanisms.

On the other hand, the physician should realize that in its initial impact a problem may be quite overpowering and some partial or initial denial is a fundamental defense mechanism. He should not interfere with this, nor with the occasional rest periods during the adaptation process when the patient tries for a while to forget his problems by diverting his interest to other matters. In fact the physician who knows his patient may be able to recognize when he is becoming too fatigued by facing the unfaceable, and he may then prescribe a temporary respite by diversion or drugs. He should be on the alert, however, to call a return to the fray once the rest period has resulted in the replenishment of resources.

I would like to sound here a word of warning against the indiscriminate and continuous use of tranquilizing drugs for people in crisis. Studies are at present under way to determine not only their pharmacophysical ill effects but also their possible psychological complications; among the latter I predict we will probably find that, by damping down too drastically the impact of crisis situations, tranquilizers may be preventing the active processes of healthy adaptation to important life difficulties and thus laying the stage for subsequent psychiatric illness.

Need for Psychiatric Consultation

The family physician who seriously wishes to enlarge the scope of his practical operations in order to cater to the mental health needs of his patients and their families would be well advised to build up a collaborative working relationship with a psychiatrist of his choice. If a psychiatrist is not available, such help can also be obtained from a well-trained clinical psychologist or a psychiatric social worker. The important thing is wherever possible to use the same person each time, so that the two can learn each other's language and ways of working.

In talking about consultation I do not have in mind the occasional necessity to refer a patient with some psychiatric illness to a specialist for investigation and treatment. This will certainly be necessary, and the more sophisticated the family physician becomes in dealing with emotional problems in his patients the earlier he will be able to identify such conditions and the more easily and surely he will be able to effect the referral procedure.

More Effective Understanding and Management

The kind of consultation I am particularly referring to here is different: it is consultation by the general physician with the psychiatric specialist in order to enlist the latter's help in rendering the family physician's own understanding of the case and his own management of it more effective.

However well trained the general physician may be, he will inevitably come across situations involving the emotional life of his patients which are outside the area of his previous learning and experience. The psychiatrist may, by discussing the case with him, be able to enlarge his understanding and to deepen his insight by pointing to the relevance of certain items of information about the field of forces which the physician had previously ignored. The psychiatrist's specialized knowledge of patterns of intrapsychic functioning and unconscious motivation may allow him to explain previously puzzling aspects of the patient's personality and that of his relatives which throw new light on their behavior and afford new opportunities for helpful action by the physician. It is very important for the doctor to tailor his intervention in the family to the special individual personality characteristics of its members. Most family physicians will build up a store of relevant knowledge of the weaknesses and strengths of their patients from their years of experience with them, but every now and again there will be some reactions which are quite unexpected and the physician may find his best efforts frustrated. On such occasions the psychiatrist's knowledge of the deeper unconscious aspects of personality functioning may clarify the situation so that the physician may find a new way to help his patient.

Improving Use of the Self

Another type of help which the physician may expect from the mental health consultation is that of sharpening and improving his own use of the self in his professional medical functioning. A physician constantly makes use of different aspects of his personal influence on his patients as part and parcel of his daily work. This use of the effect of one human being who is being helpful on another who is in need becomes especially important in dealing with those needs which are predominantly emotional rather than physicial.

Unfortunately, although physicians make use of personal influence all the time in their medical practice, this usually remains an amateur, somewhat haphazard set of operations with most physicians rather than a consciously directed professional therapeutic instrument. Some physicians have a more consistently therapeutic personal effect on patients than others, and we ascribe this to innate personality gifts or to a generalized "bedside manner" of uncertain origin. Even these physicians often fail in their efforts to support or stimulate or reassure certain patients, and when they fail they can no more understand why this has happened and deal with the consequences than they can understand their successful cases. The average physician is no better off when it comes to understanding his own special emotional reactions to certain patients—his feelings of liking and warm protectiveness, his irritability and anger, his frustration, his anxiety, or sometimes his guilty withdrawal. He does his best to control these feelings and not allow them to interfere with his objective medical approach, and his training usually helps him to succeed—but often at the expense of becoming rather distant and cold. It is the rare general physician who is able to capitalize consciously, both for diagnostic and for therapeutic purposes, on his awareness of his own feelings as they are stimulated by the behavior of his patient.

The psychiatrist, on the other hand, has by a long and arduous training not only learned to know and accept his own human reactions in his reciprocal interaction with his patients but he has learned to make explicit and differentiated use of them in the professional setting. Through the consultation process the physician may gain from him some understanding and skill in this matter. This will only come gradually, which is another reason for working with the same consultant over a lengthy period. This is not a matter of the giving or the receiving of intellectual prescriptions but the emotional education which comes from numerous discussions about the details of practical life situations and one's feelings about them.

Consultation, a Two-Way Process

So far I have talked as though the psychiatrist were the teacher and the family physician the pupil in the consultations, and to some extent this is so; but the physician who imagines that all he will have to do is to ask questions and get the answers from the psychiatrist will be sadly disappointed. He will quickly discover that with all his specialized knowledge the psychiatrist does not have many answers to the circumscribed questions about the practical issues of management of ordinary patients in the situation of general practice.

I said before that mental health consultation is a joint collaborative endeavor, and what I meant to imply is that it has to be a two-way process, in which not only the psychiatrist but also the physician must be an active partner. It is essential for the physician to realize that he must take active steps to educate the psychiatrist during these consultations so that he will understand the special nature of the management problems involved, which will be quite different from what he is used to in the very unusual circumstances of his psychiatric clinic or office practice. Working with the same psychiatrist over a period of time the physician may be able to teach him enough about the daily problems of general practice and the life situations of ordinary people who do not consider themselves psychiatric patients that he can eventually get answers which come reasonably close to being useful, but he will usually have to work quite actively to take what the psychiatrist has to offer and to translate it for his own use.

A psychiatrist who has himself had experience in general practice before undergoing psychiatric training sometimes finds this type of consultation easier, but it is surprising how specialized psychiatric training and experience, which dwell constantly on the abnormal and the unusual and on unconscious motivation and irrational fantasy formation, impair the memories of this previous experience with the world of normality. A psychiatrist usually realizes the extent to which this is so and realizes and respects the degree of expertness of the family doctor's specialized knowledge in his own field only after he has been educated by his consultee.

I can vouch personally for the importance of this process because in the course of my own experience in community psychiatry I have been successively educated by social workers, public health nurses, pediatricians, obstetricians, and nutritionists, most of whom were initially a little suprised to find how much they were teaching me during their consultations.

Responsibility for Plan and Implementation
This leads me to my last point. The management plan which emerges from the consultation may have been arrived at as a result of a fruitful joint collaborative endeavor, but the type of plan and the responsibility for its implementation must remain with the family physician and must fit into the general framework of his traditional methods of functioning. Both parties should beware of working out a psychiatrist's plan instead of a family physician's plan and of turning the physician into a "proxy psychiatrist." The style of work of the family physician is fundamentally different from that of the psychiatrist.

For instance, take the time relations of their professional work. It may seem that a busy general practitioner would never have the time to make use of the kind of knowledge I have been discussing in this paper; he could never spend the time which the psychiatrist can apparently allot to his small select group of patients. This is a red herring. It presupposes that, to cover the same problem, members of the two professional disciplines will use the same approach. This is neither necessary nor desirable, since the different professional roles have been differentiated over a long time in order to cope with problems in a very special way which has been found empirically to be effective and which is recognized by being embodied in the traditional culture of that profession. In this case, for instance, the practices of the psychiatrist in relation to time are based on the fact that his patients are strangers to him; since he has to penetrate below their surface defenses and deal with unrecognized and unacceptable material, his relationship with his patient, however intimate the content of their discussions, remains a highly structured stranger relationship, in which each takes care to keep outside the boundaries of each other's customary social life. The regular appointment and the 50-minute hour are derivatives of this situation, the interview between patient and psychiatrist being specially separated from the rest of the patient's life so as to give him the security to lay down temporarily some of his defenses. The length of the usual psychotherapeutic treatment is also dictated by the fact that the psychiatrist has to deal systematically with much complicated material in working down from the surface of consciousness to those hidden areas in which he searches for the unconscious sources of the illness.

The family physician by contrast knows many of his

patients as friends. He has known them and their relatives for years, and even in the case of a new patient he can assume that this will be a prolonged contact. He does not need to collect important information about the personality of his patients in a few long highly structured interviews; it comes in dribs and drabs, either directly or indirectly from many and various collateral sources. He penetrates the patient's social life and home as a friend, and very often his patients come into his own home as a friend. Certainly he learns many secret and intimate things about his patients, but the level of such knowledge and the confidence in professional secrecy are such that this rarely leads to a patient feeling the need to hide from the physician in social situations.

Finally, one must realize that, in helping his patient handle emotional problems of the crisis type I have referred to, the family physician does not need to make long speeches. The most powerful interpersonal messages in which one person influences another are often very short. When the time is ripe at the height of the crisis, the right word or the right few words in the right place give better results than a lecture. Often it is a brief aside or an implication of some statement which ostensibly deals with some detail of management of a physical symptom which does the trick. Very often the most powerful messages are conveyed without words—by one's understanding manner, by one's patience, by one's warmth of greeting, or by a sympathetic nod or gesture. These do not take time, and these are the stock in trade of the physician. The results will be determined by their appropriateness in relation to the specific condition of the patient in his current predicament; but if success is only partial the family physician can always rely on being able to wait for additional opportunities in the future, since his relation with his patient will probably be continuing for many years to come. Through his consultations with the psychiatrist, he will gradually become more and more skillful in these areas. I believe that this skill is a main prerequisite for success in preventing emotional illness in our communities.

References

Bowlby, J. *Maternal care and mental health. World Health Organization monograph*, 1951, Series 2.

Caplan, G. Disturbance of mother-child relationships by unsuccessful attempts at abortion. *Mental Hygiene*, 1954, 38, 670-680.

Caplan, G. Psychological aspects of maternity care. *American Journal of Public Health*, 1957, 47, 25-31.

Lindemann, E. Symptomatology and management of acute grief. *American Journal of Psychiatry*, 1944, 101, 141-148.

7

The Contribution of School to Personality Development*

When I first met Bill Cannon, we spent most of our time discussing ways of improving the care of emotionally disturbed students in the Boston School Department, and what emerged were the foundations of our Harvard Mental Health Program in the schools. As time passed, however, we talked of more fundamental issues; and I realized that he was not only a highly competent educator and administrator, but also a man with lively intellectual curiosity about the borderland between education and psychology. He was willing to think innovatively about ways of improving schooling so that all students, not just the emotionally disturbed, might develop stronger and more resilient personalities. His mental flexibility and courage in crossing accepted boundaries of thought and professional functioning did much to stimulate me to consider these questions: How can we organize a school so that it provides the best supportive structure within which students can develop healthy personalities? What is the importance of order and discipline in such a school? How is this related to the complex environment of which the

*The First Annual William L. Cannon Memorial Lecture, Jimmy Fund Bldg., Boston School Dept. Boston, April 16, 1970.

educational system is only a part? In a rapidly changing world, should our curriculum focus explicitly on current events and be seen by the students to be directly relevant to their present concerns? What should be the responsibility of the educator in deciding what is relevant? How can the educator help his students prepare for the unexpected problems of life? How can he ensure that his students achieve their maximal potential? I certainly cannot hope to provide a satisfying answer to these major questions, but I hope to define some of the relevant issues.

An Arab School In Jerusalem

I have recently returned from Jerusalem where I have been studying problems of communication between Jews and Arabs. As part of my research, I investigated recent developments in the school system of the Arab population of East Jerusalem and the effects of these developments on the adjustment of teachers and students to the present situation. Just before I left Jerusalem, I visited an Arab private boys' school, and I will begin with a brief account of what I found and its significance for the topic of personality development.

The school was established 94 years ago by a French religious order which still directs it. It is housed in a series of granite buildings in the Christian Quarter just inside the medieval walls of the Old City. I visited it one rainy morning with an Arab research assistant; my first impression was of a forbidding place. The long grey stone corridors with their high vaulted roofs were strangely silent although there were 1,000 boys between the ages of five and 18 in the adjoining classrooms. In contrast with the usual Arab schools of Jerusalem, it was remarkably neat and decorous. Eventually, we reached the principal's office. At one end of this large bare room there was a huge desk, in front of which were two straight rows of upright chairs set 10 feet away. The awesome formality of the setting was accented by the fact that the only heating came from a small kerosene stove, and the room was so cold that I kept my coat on throughout the interview.

Behind the desk was the Director, a severe-looking French monk. I was somewhat nonplussed by the fact that after I had chosen a chair in the front row, there was about 14 feet of space between me and the Director; but I regained some composure when, in addition to the customary choice of coffee or tea, he added a French touch of hospitality by also offering us cognac. At nine in the morning on a cold wet Jerusalem day this might have been attractive, but I suppose I was so startled by the setting that I clung instinctively to my own cultural habits and asked for tea!

As I spoke to the Director, my surprise increased. Over the previous few weeks, I had grown familiar with the instability in many of the East Jerusalem schools which had been aggravated by the social, economic, and political changes in the city since the 1967 War. In contrast, this school had had no significant turnover of staff or students. The traditions were kept unchanged—children are only admitted at kindergarten level, because, as the Director said, "We need students who have acquired our spirit of working hard, and we cannot inculcate this unless we get children at the beginning of their school career." He told me that by and large he admits only the sons of alumni, or boys whose older brothers were already enrolled. Thus a family tradition of hard work and discipline is developed.

The Director was very proud of the discipline in his school, and I began to feel sorry for the boys who were condemned to this cold, rigid, and authoritarian atmosphere. I did not ask whether corporal punishment was used. It was clear that the threat of being sent to that principal's office to be admonished or, even worse, of being suspended or expelled from the school at which your brothers, your father, and possibly your grandfather had studied, was a more potent factor than the fear of temporary pain. As the interview progressed, my assessment of the strict authoritarianism of the school did not change, but I gradually began to have doubts about its negative impact on the students.

The Director told me that about two-thirds of his students were Christians and about one third were Moslems. "Of course," he said, "we forbid all discussion of religion and politics, on pain of expulsion, but I have never been forced to expel any boy for disobeying this fundamental rule. We also allow no discussion of the war with Israel. Our task is education; and whatever the world is like outside, within these walls our students and teachers focus all energy on studying our curriculum. The more uncertain the world into which our students will graduate, the more they need a disciplined mind and a good academic knowledge so as to find their own way." This led us into a discussion of the psychological reactions of his students, and he told me that he had long been impressed by the necessity for an educator not only to develop the policies and curriculum of his school in order to provide an atmosphere conducive to good academic work habits in the total population of students, but also to focus particular attention on individual children who for a variety of reasons might have difficulties in progressing. He believed that family influences were most important here; and he had developed a system of regular and close communication between teachers and parents, both to ensure steady parental pressure on their children to conform to school demands and also to detect and remedy tensions within the family that might interfere with a child's capacity to learn. The Director held office hours twice a week for parents; and he said, "The most important part of my job is the counselling I give parents about home problems that have an effect on their children." When I asked for examples, he told me of recent cases of marital disharmony in which he had intervened—in one case even calling in and admonishing a father whose wife had complained to him that her husband was being unfaithful. When I expressed some surprise at such an extension of his educational role, he told me that the father, as is not unusual in that school, had in the past been a student of his, and so continued to have a special relationship to him as a wise authority figure.

The Director felt that the educator's role as a counsellor relates not only to family conflicts but also to psychological upheavals of individual children, particularly during adolescence. He emphasized the opportunities for counselling and psychological support in his school because it was organized by a religious Brotherhood. Of the 42 teachers in the school, 10 were monks; they formed a kind of family group whose doors were always open to any student who wanted to enter at a time of crisis, during or after school hours or during vacations. Many students used this opportunity and developed personal relationships with one or more of the Brothers, to whom they turned for counsel either about personal matters or about problems in their studies or careers. Thus, it became clear that although authority in the school is strict, it is also solicitous, and that the Director and his teachers are probably seen by their students as a devoted group of wise and disciplined adults who care deeply about them.

I intend to revisit this school next time I go to

Jerusalem in order to explore it further; meanwhile, my observations suggest the following ideas:

A Structured Haven
In a tumultuous, rapidly changing, crisis-ridden world, school can successfully provide a haven of structure, order, and stability which permits the child to acquire capabilities for problem-solving and facilitates personal development.

Discipline and Autonomy
Personal autonomy depends on internal discipline, and one way of achieving this is for the child to conform to a disciplined social structure during the school years. One effective way of organizing a disciplined school is through the adult authority of the educators, who create a network of expectations among the students and their families that this is necessary and good. If such traditions are maintained, individual deviance is likely to be minimal.

Support and Guidance
General control of behavior and academic pressure may be necessary, but are not sufficient to foster individual competence and autonomy. They must be supplemented by support and guidance for the many individuals who have difficulty in conforming to the group norms. Counselling of students and families should be provided by educators who are perceived to care for and understand their students. The educators should be available during times of crisis and should be alert for signs that a particular student is beginning to show evidence of strain. This will probably be manifested in reduced classroom performance or in difficulties with other students, but will often be related to problems in the home or in other

aspects of the child's private life, such as intra-psychic conflicts of adolescence.

Values and Models

Healthy personality development requires not only the acceptance of external discipline that is eventually internalized, but also the development of values and a style of behavior to guide one's striving. These are mainly acquired by identification with role models—admired and respected adults or peers. The capacity to be such a model is the supreme challenge for the educator. To some extent, how he handles this depends on his basic personality, but he also needs support from the organization of the school to maintain his own poise. In our example, the small cohesive group of Brothers probably provides such mutual support, and their religious vocation is an important factor. In other schools this support must come from the leadership of the principal and the development of satisfying relationships within the staff group.

Loving acceptance is a necessity for healthy personality development. In our culture this should be found in the family circle. What is provided in the family can be effectively augmented, and sometimes if necessary replaced, by the individualized solicitude of an educator.

Relevance

What does our example teach us about the importance of relevance of curriculum content to the problems of the real world? Apparently, it refutes the current popular belief that this is supremely important. The curriculum in that Jerusalem school is deliberately divorced from the ethnic, religious, and political problems of the world outside the school walls. It has nevertheless been found most acceptable by the local Arab population. They do not even appear to have objected to the curriculum being geared to a final examination—the London General College Entrance Examination—set by a culture at the other side of the world, whose consonance with the Arab way of life and the economy of Jerusalem is doubtful. In fact, many of the school's graduates have left home to study in foreign universities and eventually have emigrated because they have not been able to adjust to the conditions of their local society.

In order to understand this paradox we should consider four important aspects of relevance:

First, relevance signifies that the education fits the child to play his part in the present or future life of his own or a foreign community.

Second, the curriculum may focus directly on the outside world, or it may be linked to it abstractly by inculcating theoretical principles and spiritual values derived from studying issues far removed in space and time, like the literature of ancient Rome. These principles will enable the student to find his own way in dealing with the complexities of his life when the need arises.

Third, the student's belief that a curriculum is relevant may derive from his own assessment of its links with the real world, or else from his accepting testimony to this effect from parents and teachers. The degree to which a student pays attention to the views of the adults will depend on the quality of the relationship of trust and respect between the generations.

Fourth, the conviction that the curriculum is relevant, however it is derived, exerts a major influence on a student's motivation to learn. He will tend to mobilize effort and to overcome obstacles only to the degree that he believes that he is being asked to study something useful.

In the Jerusalem school it seems that, although the curriculum might not be evaluated by an objective outsider to have proved relevant either to the present or future demands of the city and the country, it has been chosen by the French educators to fit their own view of a universalistic standard of academic excellence that transcends the needs of a particular locality. The Arab parents, who have mixed feelings about living in a city with poor resources, have probably been satisfied, in part, because the school equips its students to seek a better life in the wider Arab world or in the West. The most important factor, however, is that in their traditional society acceptance of authority is automatic. The parents therefore conform to the will of the teachers, and the children in turn rely on the judgment of their parents. The students do not think of questioning the curriculum, and their motivation to learn is, therefore, not weakened by analyzing its present or future lack of relevance.

The Effects of Changing Values

However, the Middle East has recently been moving toward social revolution. The old order is beginning to change, and, particularly in Jerusalem, the traditional values of the Arabs are being shaken by contact with the open society of the Israelis. It is therefore likely that in the near future Jerusalem Arab parents may begin to question the long term effects of this educational system that drives away the best of their children, or that gluts the market of a relatively poorly developed country with a white collar and intellectual class destined for chronic frustration because appropriate local job opportunities commensurate with their academic level and career aspirations are not available. The students, too, may begin to think for themselves. When that happens, the system in the Jerusalem school may well begin to break down, and its educators may no longer be free to determine how and what to teach to whom because they will have lost the unquestioning acceptance by the students and their parents of their unilateral right to make the fundamental educational decisions.

It is this kind of upset in the established order of trust and dependency between parents and educators and between youth and adults that is responsible for much of the educational turmoil in our part of the world. In the consequent confusion, educators sometimes have the tendency to throw the baby out with the bathwater. Because our traditional authority is now being seriously and vociferously questioned, some of us begin to abdicate our responsibility and to opt for a quieter life by handing over the power to decide what and how to teach entirely to our students. Relevance then becomes a matter for students to decide in line with their current interests. Instead, responsible educators argue that even if they no longer are given the unquestioned authority of the Director of that Jerusalem school, they should nevertheless exercise their specialized competence in planning an appropriate curriculum, while also taking into account the power and significance of the attitudes and ideas of students and parents.

The wise educator who still retains unquestioned right to make fundamental educational decisions for his students has a special freedom to innovate in areas that he deems important. The Director of the Jerusalem school, for example, told me that he was no longer completely satisfied with the classroom as a medium for educational influence, especially in preparing his students for social competence. He was, therefore, experimenting with extra-curricular activities and had fostered a series of student clubs dealing with such issues as music, art, and cultural affairs. Some of the student clubs were beginning to explore the life of West Jerusalem and were initiating contacts with Israeli children and cultural institutions. I was here reminded of the work of Kurt Hahn (1957), in Salem, Germany, after the First World War, and later, following the rise of Hitler, in Britain, where he established the private school at Gordonstoun that has become famous as the place where the Prince of Wales was educated. Prince Philip, the Duke of Edinburgh, had been educated at Kurt Hahn's school in Salem, as were the sons of several of the other noble families of Europe.

I first met Kurt Hahn when he asked my help in assessing the mental health implications of his educational pioneering. I discovered that for some years he had been preoccupied by the problem of how to make the results of his researches into the education of the children of the rich and famous available to ordinary people. He had thus developed the Outward Bound movement with which some of you may be familiar, and which became one of the models for our own Peace Corps.

Hahn's basic assumption is that it is the task of the educator to stimulate and support his students in extending their interests and personal skills beyond the boundaries of their current concepts and beliefs in their own capacities. His attitude to a student's ideas on relevance is unequivocal. He says, "If a student comes to me who is an introvert, I influence him to become outgoing. If he is interested in science, I satisfy that interest but I open his eyes also to art and humanities." In other words, Hahn takes it upon himself to widen and deepen his student's ideas on what is relevant. Like the Director of the Jerusalem school, he does not only focus on the present content of what is being learned, which may be all that a student might take into account in line with his current interests or with his appraisal of his daily world;

as an educator, Hahn pays attention also to the basic values and habits of mind that are being unconsciously acquired by the student at the same time: self-discipline, methodical work patterns, respect for abiding cultural and ethical values, and a perspective on daily life widened by knowledge of history and philosophy. These might in the future be judged more relevant to the real world in which that individual may find himself than the subject matter of individual courses. The ideal of such educators is that their students should acquire ways of thinking that make them self-sufficient, whatever the environment to which they will eventually be exposed.

In pursuit of this goal Hahn emphasizes extra-curricular education. He places his students in situations that are physically challenging, like mountaineering and ocean sailing, or that are socially demanding, like welfare work with deprived people of an alien culture. He believes in the fundamental urge of young people to save life and to do something meaningful for their fellow men; thus most of the extra-curricular activities he advocates are linked with rescue work, social service, or training for first aid and life saving. In such situations he exposes his students to progressively more demanding and challenging tasks, each of which is graduated to be just beyond the student's current capacity. His educators have the job of supervising this process so as to prevent the student from endangering himself or others, and of encouraging and supporting him to discover and exploit unexpected physical and moral resources in himself and others as he grapples with the obstacles he encounters. In terms of the mental health theories of our Harvard Group, Hahn precipitates in his students a series of psychosocial crises, and then helps them find healthy ways of mastering them. This results in a progressive strengthening and expansion of personality, leading not only to increased competence, but to an enlargement of the student's awareness of his own strength, and hence to improved resilience and poise. Since an individual's level of mental health is linked with his capacity to react positively to unexpected life crises, Hahn's educational approach, if it were adopted widely, would provide a means whereby we might increase the resistance to mental disorder of a large population.

Another educational researcher who has contributed to this topic is Ralph Ojemann of Iowa (1961). He, too, focuses on the goal of educating students to improve their capacity to solve unfamiliar problems. In contrast to Hahn, he seeks to achieve this inside the classroom. Ojemann criticizes both the curriculum and the style of teaching in most American schools as leading to what he calls "surface or manifestational" thinking. By this he means that students are trained to perceive a problematic issue or situation in terms of one of a series of possible patterns, to each of which there is a stereotyped appropriate response that the student must memorize. Ojemann seeks to replace this by teaching students to analyze any situation or manifestation by discovering its causal elements, and to seek the solution of problems by thinking out the effects of modifying these causal elements. He calls this "education in causal thinking." He has rewritten the curriculum content of the school program in all subjects in order to convey this message, and he has trained teachers to modify their teaching style along similar lines.

Ojemann has carried out some excellent evaluation studies of the effects on children receiving "causal" teaching as contrasted with those exposed to the more usual "manifestational" teaching. He has demonstrated that the former are more effective in solving unfamiliar problems than a matched group of the latter. One of his research findings that is most important from a mental health viewpoint is that children educated in casual thinking have an increased capacity to persevere in grappling with difficult problems in the face of confusion and frustration. Our mental health studies on reactions of individuals to crisis situations have clearly demonstrated that such perseverence is the most important factor in determining a healthy adaptive response. Once again, as with Kurt Hahn, the hope is aroused that a total population may have its level of mental health raised by improved schooling—not by reducing environmental sources of stress but by increasing the capacity of individuals to master it.

What is common to the approach both of Hahn and of Ojemann, as well as implicit in the educational philosophy of the Jerusalem school, is that the educators challenge their students by confronting them with tasks that are so difficult that they produce strain. This must be based upon the belief of the educators that their students are inherently capable of mastering such strain, at least with the guidance and support of the adults. This fundamental respect for their students' basic abilities is part of the image that the educators have of them, and some researchers have recently conducted an interesting study of the effects on the educational process and on the performance of students when an educator's image of his students is experimentally modified. Robert A. Rosenthal and Lenore Jacobsen in their recent book, *Pygmalion in the Classroom* (1968), have reported on an experiment they carried out in a California school, where they informed teachers that certain of their children had I.Q.'s higher than were being reflected in their achievement scores. The supposed "high I.Q." children were, in fact, randomly selected without relationship to their actual intelligence. The authors reported dramatic improvements in achievement of these children compared with a control group, and they attributed these to changes in teacher expectation and consequent treatment of students. Unfortunately, the quality of the research methods and the way the data were analysed in this study has been severely criticized by competent reviewers such as Thorndike (1968) and Snow (1969), and we must treat the results with caution until the study has been confirmed by other researchers.

On the other hand, the results are in line with those of several other recent studies about perceptions and expectations by teachers of children of different race and social class, and the effect of these on the teaching process and on its results. Gottlieb (1964) compared Negro and white elementary school teachers' views of their students. He found that Negro teachers in low-income areas expressed more satisfaction with their work. They tended to see their black students as fun-loving, happy, cooperative, energetic, and ambitious. White teachers perceived the same students as talkative, lazy, fun-loving, high strung, and frivolous.

A similar study by Davidson and Lang (1960) revealed that teachers generally rated classroom behavior of lower-class children as undesirable even when their academic achievements were good. Children became aware of teachers' critical attitudes and acquired lower perceptions of themselves. Deutsch (1960) has shown that such children subsequently achieve less and behave less satisfactorily because of what he terms "poor self-fulfillment prophesy."

Other studies, such as one by the New York agency, Haryou (1964), have revealed that many middle-class teachers feel that the lower class child is intellectually limited. The result of this, as shown by Silberman (1964), is that "The teacher who assumes that her children cannot learn very much will discover that she has a class of children who are indeed unable to learn."

Discussion

As I ponder the significance of the work of these pioneering educators and researchers, I begin to appreciate the constituents of the kind of school atmosphere that influences the personality of students. In trying to communicate my impressions of the Jerusalem school I found myself describing its physical characteristics, such as the stone of which it is constructed, and temperature of the Director's office, and the seating arrangements of his room. I also included in my description apparently irrelevant personal matters, such as my own lack of poise when confronting the Director, and his strict appearance and manner. All of these details, and many more, turned out to be not at all irrelevant, but to add up to an impression that conveyed to me, and I hope to you, a very definite but quite complicated message. I imagine it communicates most powerfully a similar message to the students—not in any set of explicit words and not in a way that might be obvious to them or to a casual observer, but by the underlying feeling. The very walls of the school, its internal structure and the manner and bearing of its personnel form a consistent nonverbal pattern that impresses itself on the students.

Closer to home, many of our students demand as their price for participation in the educational process not only that the educator should fit in with their wish that what he teaches should seem currently relevant to them, but also that the formal aspects of the school milieu should fit their immediate needs for comfort, diversion, and relaxation. They may be supported in this demand by their parents in the name of "progressive education" where learning is supposed to be fun, or because the parents wish to evade the difficulty of dealing with their rebellious progeny by a laissez-faire approach, taking the line of least resistance.

If educators are not careful, a school milieu may be created that is comfortable and free from tension, both academic and disciplinary, but which unfortunately, also conveys a false nonverbal message: that life rewards wish-fulfilling fantasies, that complicated problems can best be handled by quick solutions, that frustration and confusion should signal immediate evasion of the stressful issue, that order and attention to detail are of no importance, or that adults really do not care for the young and are prepared to give in to their inconsistent demands whenever they make sufficient noise. This path clearly leads not just to comfortable chaos, but to inevitable future frustration and anxiety in the students and to the apathy of impotence in the adults, as well as to the promotion of optimal conditions for weak personality development and impaired mental health of all concerned.

On the other hand, since our present disequilibrated society does not provide our educators with the easy framework within which the traditional educators worked, how can we avoid this unfortunate path? I have no ready answer, except to say that this is a field where it would seem profitable for educators and mental health specialists to work together in search of new ways of securing the concurrence of students and parents to the organizing of schools that prepare students to master the expectable problems of life by mobilizing effort, rather than to evade them and to release tension. I believe that educators and mental health workers should combine to define the essential elements of a desirable educational milieu and to communicate this to community leaders and to influential parents so as to elicit their support, not in the name of tradition, but because it makes sense on the basis of empirical experience and the findings of scientific researchers. Such a list of essential elements might include the following:

Structure
The physical and social structure of the school should communicate to the students that life will probably present them with difficult problems and challenges that they must learn to master.

Mastery
Mastery may come in two ways: One can learn what problems to expect and how to go about solving them, or one can learn how to wrestle with unexpected problems. The latter involves understanding the basic principles of problem solving and learning how to persevere despite confusion and frustration.

Guidance and Support
Students should be helped to learn how to mobilize unexpected sources of strength in themselves and others in dealing with problems. Educators should provide guidance and support directly and should also stimulate students to ask for help and provide help to others within their peer group.

Discipline
Effective problem solving demands an orderly and systematic individual approach as well as assurance of social support from peers, subordinates and superiors. This psychological structure is internalized after repeatedly experiencing similar patterns in the operations of the school. Order and discipline, as well as consistency of social behavior, are therefore of great importance.

Role Models

The values of the culture should be communicated not only explicitly in verbal formulations but by the implications of everyday behavior in the school community. Of particular importance is the function of the educators as role models.

Morale

Leadership and good interpersonal relationships in the group of educators must ensure their high morale, because the quality of this morale will have a major influence upon the student body. This implies careful selection of educators and good personnel practices.

Communication

What binds the students and educators together as individuals and groups is the network of their mutual expectations. Irrational distortions based on racial and social prejudice or ignorance will upset the cohesion of this system of bonds. Special mechanisms, such as regular staff conferences, supervision, mental health consultation, and informal meetings between teachers and students should be developed to identify and remedy such distortions.

All such mechanisms depend upon opening up communication so that reality-based information may be conveyed in order to dissipate stereotyped perceptions and expectations.

Problem-Solving

Education in solving problems and in improving the students' capacities for self-mastery should take place not only in the classroom but also in extra-curricular activities outside the school buildings. The latter aspect of education demands adequate budget and staff, and it should be regarded as an essential part of schooling.

Education for Leisure

Students should be educated not only for the serious side of life but also to express themselves socially and artistically so that they learn how to fulfill themselves in interpersonal and leisure activities. They must learn how to safely and constructively relax and enjoy themselves. Here, too, the educators should act as role models, and the school should provide opportunities for teachers and students to join in the enjoyment of leisure.

Inclusion of Deviant Subgroups

The social and physical structure of the school caters to the total population of students and necessarily must adopt a standardized pattern and a set of expectable norms. The structure should also include facilities and programs for dealing with deviant subgroups and individuals, such as slow learners and children who for family and individual psychological reasons have short or long term difficulty in adjusting. They should have opportunities for privacy, for temporary withdrawal from the hurly-burly of the general student body. Staff time should be budgeted and personnel should be given appropriate specialized training, supervision and consultation, so that in such instances individually tailored counselling or tuition can be made freely available whenever it is needed.

Time does not permit me to add to this list, which is clearly far from complete. It does, however, give some indication of what I have in mind, and perhaps it offers one approach that might turn out to be of value in grappling with a major issue of our day and age.

References

Davidson, H. K. & Lang, G. Children's perceptions of their teachers' feelings toward them related to self-perception, school achievement and behavior. *Journal of Experimental Education*, 1960, 29, 107-118.

Deutsch, M. *Minority group and class status as related to social and personality factors in scholastic achievement. Society for Applied Anthropology Monographs*, New York: Cornell University, 1960, No. 2.

Gottlieb, D. Teaching and students: The views of negro and white teachers, *Sociology and Education*, 1964, 37, 345-53.

Hahn, K. The origins of the Outward Bound trust. In D. James (Ed.), *Outward Bound*. London: Routeledge and Kegan Paul, 1957. Pp. 1-18.

Haryou, Inc. *Youth in the ghetto: A study of the consequence of powerlessness and a blueprint for change*. New York: Haryou, Inc., 1964.

Ojemann, R. H. Investigations on the effects of teaching an understanding and appreciation of behavior dynamics. In G. Caplan (Ed.), *Prevention of mental disorders in children*. New York: Basic Books, 1961. Pp. 378-398.

Rosenthal, R. & Jacobsen, L. *Pygmalion in the classroom*. New York: Rinehart & Winston, 1968.

Silberman, C. E. *Crisis in black and white*. New York: Vintage Books, 1964.

Snow, R. L. Unfinished pygmalion. Review of R. Rosenthal & L. Jacobsen, *Pygmalion in the classroom. Contemporary Psychology*, 1969, 14, 197-199.

Thorndike, R. L. Review of R. Rosenthal & L. Jacobsen, *Pygmalion in the classroom. American Educational Research Journal*, 1968, 5, 708-711.

8

Preventing Mental Disorders*

In recent years we have begun to realize that mental disorders are so numerous that our traditional psychiatric treatment services can never hope to deal with more than a fraction of the cases which occur.

A current survey in Boston by Ryan (1962) reveals that out of every 1000 persons in the population, more than 150 have been identified by community professionals as significantly handicapped because of emotional disturbance. Only 10 of this 150 get help in a mental health setting: five go to a mental hospital, four receive treatment in a mental health clinic for adults or children, and one is treated by a psychiatrist in private practice. Of the remaining 140, about 60 are cared for by physicians in private practice or in general hospitals. Another 10 are handled by casework agencies, settlement houses, and churches. The remainder are not being specifically helped by any professional resource.

This sorry state of affairs is not confined to Boston, which in fact has a better developed network of psychiatric services than many other cities, and is immeasurably better than most rural areas. For instance, the states of Alaska, Wyoming, Idaho, Nevada, and Montana have less than 20 psychiatrists each.

*A lecture delivered at The Modern Forum, Los Angeles, California, on December 5, 1964.

Our national leaders have begun to face up to this situation. In 1955, Congress created the Joint Commission on Mental Illness and Health to study the problem. In 1961 the Commission published its report, Action For Mental Health. In February, 1963, the late President Kennedy, after studying this report, sent a message to Congress which enunciated the policy of his Administration. He said:

> Mental illness and mental retardation are among our most critical health problems. They occur more frequently, affect more people, require more prolonged treatment, cause more suffering by the families of the afflicted, waste more of our human resources, and constitute more financial drain upon both the Public Treasury and the personal finances of the individual families than any other single condition. . . . This situation has been tolerated far too long. . . . The time has come for a bold new approach. . . . Governments at every level—Federal, State, and local—private foundations and individual citizens must all face up to their responsibilities in this area. . . . Our attack must be focused on three major objectives:
>
> First, we must seek out the causes of mental illness and of mental retardation and eradicate them. Here more than in any other area, "an ounce of prevention is worth more than a pound of cure." For prevention is far more desirable for all concerned. It is far more economical and it is far more likely to be successful. Prevention will require both selected specific programs directed especially at known causes, and the general strengthening of our fundamental community, social welfare, and educational programs which can do much to eliminate or correct the harsh en-

vironmental conditions which often are associated with mental retardation and mental illness. . . .

Second, we must strengthen the underlying resources of knowledge, and, above all, of skilled manpower which are necessary to mount and sustain our attack on mental disability for many years to come. . . .

Third, we must strengthen and improve the programs and facilities serving the mentally ill and the mentally retarded. . . . Services to both the mentally ill and to the mentally retarded must be community based and provide a range of services to meet community needs. . . .

I propose a national mental health program to assist in the inauguration of a wholly new emphasis and approach to care for the mentally ill.

Eight months later, on October 31, 1963, Congress enacted legislation which authorized federal matching funds of $150 million for use over three years by the states in constructing comprehensive community mental health centers which will be designed to implement the program advocated by President Kennedy.

In this chapter I will discuss the preventive services which will be an integral part of this program, and which President Kennedy singled out as its first and most important component.

Types of Prevention

Preventive psychiatry can be considered under three main headings:

Primary prevention aims at reducing the incidence of new cases of mental disorder in the population by combating harmful forces which operate in the community and by strengthening the capacity of people to withstand stress. This is the type of prevention to which President Kennedy referred in his message to Congress.

Secondary prevention aims at reducing the duration of cases of mental disorder which occur in spite of the programs of primary prevention. By shortening the duration of existing cases, the prevalence of mental disorder in the community is reduced. This is accomplished by organizing case-finding, diagnostic, and remedial services so that mental disorders are detected early and are dealt with effectively. Because of the large numbers of cases and our relatively small resources of specialized workers and facilities, this means finding out how to use the specialists most productively, and how to maximize the efforts of the nonspecialized workers who will inevitably be caring for the majority of the sufferers.

Tertiary prevention aims at reducing the community rate of residual defect which is a sequel to mental disorder. It seeks to ensure that people who have recovered from mental disorder will be hampered as little as possible by their past difficulties in returning to full participation in the occupational and social life of the community. It achieves this goal by combating alienation from work, family, and social groups during and after mental illness, and by organizing programs to rehabilitate all expatients; thus parallel with the reduction of their symptoms as a consequence of therapy they will also be helped to recover their old occupational and social skills, or to acquire new ones, to the limit of their residual capacities.

All three types of preventive psychiatry focus on the total population and seek to reduce the community rates of mental disorder and its effects. This is the new approach, as advocated by President Kennedy. It contrasts with our old approach which provided therapists and institutions whose responsibility was restricted to their individual patients. The new programs are just as much interested in all those people who do not come for psychiatric help. For example, in relation to the Boston survey, preventive psychiatry is interested not only in the 10 cases currently treated by the mental health services, but also in the other 140, some of whom are cared for by other health and welfare workers and some of whom receive no professional assistance. It is also interested in the life conditions of the remaining 850 people who have not been professionally identified as mentally disordered. Some of these may have been sick in the past and may now no longer be in contact with helping agencies, but may be operating well below their optimal potential. Tertiary preventive services are interested in them. Some would probably be recognized to be suffering from early or mild disorders if they were seen by a professional worker. This is the domain of secondary prevention. Some are currently not sick but may be living in such circumstances that they are headed for future mental disorder. Programs of primary prevention are interested in them.

In order to encompass the total population a complicated set of professional and citizen activities must be organized, and there must be a planned program in the mental health field in which the deployment of specialized resources must be carefully related to a wide focus without spreading the specialists so thin that their efforts are wasted. This program must use a significant portion of the time of the mental health specialists to optimize the operations of those other workers in the health and welfare fields who currently care for the majority of the mentally disordered; and the mental health program must coordinate its operations with other programs in the community which modify the conditions of life of its citizens. Community planning, organization, and coordination are clearly fundamental elements of preventive psychiatry. This was indicated in President Kennedy's message, and is spelled out in some detail in the Federal regulations (1963) governing the utilization of funds made available by the subsequent legislation.

Primary Prevention

Primary prevention deals with the conditions of life of the currently healthy population. It deals with significant issues in the whole field of community activity—in the economic, political, occupational, public health, religious, welfare, and educational spheres. It is potentially the most attractive and most effective approach to a radical solution of the problem of mental disorder in our communities. The remainder of the chapter will focus on this type of preventive psychiatry, although I must emphasize that an adequately balanced community program must also devote significant resources to the other two types.

Primary prevention operates by modifying the population-wide patterns of forces which influence the lives of people so as to reduce the risk of their becoming mentally disordered.

Although we currently have little definite knowledge of specific factors which are conducive to particular mental disorders, we do have an increasing body of plausible assumptions about generally harmful and helpful influences. Some of these assumptions are based on clinical experience derived from seeing regularities in the histories of psychiatric patients, some are inferred from theoretical notions, some are based upon the good results of therapy which attacks specific factors, and a few are derived from epidemiologic studies which demonstrate the existence of different sets of conditions in communities which have high rates of mental disorder (as contrasted with comparison groups which have low rates of the same disorder).

In order to deal systematically with this subject preventive psychiatrists have developed a conceptual framework which helps them order these ideas. According to this model, the rates of mental disorders in a community are related to the operation of both long term and short term factors impinging on its members.

On a long term basis, the likelihood of mental disorder is felt to be increased if specified basic supplies are not adequately provided for the population. These supplies can be classified as physical, psychosocial, and sociocultural. A program of primary prevention seeks to list these supplies and to ensure their optimal provision in the population.

The short term focus of the preventive model is on the patterns of adaptation of people to developmental and situational life crises. It seems that the rate and direction of a person's psychological development throughout life, whether towards mental health or mental disorder, is increased at times of crisis. These crises represent transition points, at each of which the person may move nearer or further away from the pattern of functioning which we call mental disorder. Primary prevention seeks to reduce the intensity of crises among members of a population in order to increase their spontaneous chances of healthy adaptation. It also provides preparation before and help during crises so that a healthy outcome may be more likely.

The Nature of Long Term Supplies

Physical supplies include food, shelter, sensory stimulation, opportunities for exercise, and the like, which are necessary for bodily growth and development and for the maintenance of bodily health upon which mental health is dependent, as well as protection from bodily damage before and after birth, such as that by infection, trauma, or chemical poisons.

Psychosocial supplies include the stimulation of a person's intellectual and emotional development through personal interaction with significant other people in the family and with peers and older persons in school, church, and work. In the face-to-face interchanges the person satisfies his needs for love and affection, for limitation and control, and for participation in joint activity which provides opportunities for identification and identity formation. Inadequate provision of psychosocial supplies, which is conducive to mental disorder, occurs if there is no opportunity for a person to build relationships with others who can satisfy his needs, for instance, if he does not have a stable family; if the significant other people do not satisfy his needs but manipulate him in order to satisfy theirs, as when there is a disorder in the relationships his parents have towards him; or if satisfactory relationships are interrupted through illness, death, departure, or disillusionment.

Sociocultural supplies include those influences on personality development and functioning which are exerted by the customs and values of the culture and the social structure. The expectations by others of a person's behavior have a profound influence on his actions and on his feelings about himself. They fix his place in the structure of his society, and to a considerable degree they determine his path in life. This provides him with rewards and external security to supplement inner strength. If a person happens to be born into an advantaged group in a stable society, his social roles and their expected changes over a lifetime will provide him with adequate opportunities for healthy personality development. If, on the other hand, he belongs to a disadvantaged group or an unstable society, he may find his progress blocked, and he may be deprived of challenge and opportunity. This will have a negative effect on his mental health.

Improving the Provision of Long-Term Supplies

A program of primary prevention will survey the provision of supplies to its population and will then attempt to improve this situation—usually by modifying community-wide practices through altering laws, regulations, administrative patterns, or widespread values and attitudes.

The following examples are illustrative:

Physical Supplies

Mental disorders caused by lead poisoning in slum children, due to their eating lead paint off the decaying woodwork, are not uncommon. They could be prevented by compelling landlords to replace old paint containing lead with the modern lead-free variety.

In certain parts of this country, endemic cretinism which causes mental retardation is due to a deficiency of iodine in the drinking water. This disorder has been prevented by a regulation which has introduced iodides into table salt.

Psychoses due to pellagra caused by vitamin B deficiency have been much reduced in the southern part of the United States. Social policies and community education programs have fostered changes in the food habits and the food supplies of the population, so there is now an adequate intake of vitamin B.

A central issue in ensuring adequate physical supplies

in the population is safeguarding the bodily health of the fetus, the newborn, and the child. The preventive psychiatrist seeks to achieve this by collaborating with obstetricians, pediatricians, school health, and public health workers so that prenatal and obstetric services are utilized by more women, so that the bodily health of children and adults is fostered and supervised, and so that accidents are prevented inside the home, on the roads, in the school, and at work.

Psychosocial Supplies

A major goal is to safeguard the integrity of the family. Legislators and administrators who plan manpower distribution should be influenced to ensure that breadwinners be given work opportunities in the localities where their families live. Employment regulations covering pregnant women and mothers of young children should allow them time off to care for their children. In some countries, graduated family allowances permit mothers of young children to stay at home. Divorce laws and legal practices relating to custody of children are an important field for the consultative services of the preventive psychiatrist. In Denmark, a mental health specialist is consulted whenever a couple with children seeks a divorce; his advice influences court decisions on custody and visiting.

Illness, hospitalization, or death of the mother is a common hazard to family integrity. This often leads to fragmentation of the family, with the children being separated and sent to unstable placements with relatives or in foster homes or residential institutions. A preventive psychiatry program would help the community to provide a homemaker service so that families can be kept together in their own homes as much as possible.

Maternal deprivation due to hospitalization of a child

is a classical example of reduction of essential psychosocial supplies, as Bowlby of the Tavistock Clinic in London pointed out in 1952. This damaging factor can be combated on a community-wide scale through regulations promoting daily visiting of hospitalized children by their parents, modification of hospital structure and functioning to allow mothers to stay with and help nurse their children, and changes in the professional practice of pediatrics so that sick children are, as far as possible, treated at home and not in hospital. This also involves provision by the community of financial and home-nursing resources.

Maintaining family ties is not only important in childhood, but throughout life, and particularly in old age. Significant developments in present-day urban life are both the relative increase in the number of the aged associated with improvements in general health care, and the difficulty of maintaining regular contact between the older and younger generations because of cramped living quarters and rejecting attitudes. Preventive psychiatrists seek to influence city planners to provide more large apartments, especially in housing projects, so that grandparents need not be pushed out of the family home. Planners can also be counseled to build special housing for the aged in relatively small units spread throughout the community, so that old people can live near their children and grandchildren, and so that continuing links between them can be fostered. It is also possible to combat the attitudes of rejection of the aged by programs of public education which help younger people understand the problems and potentials of their parents and grandparents in much the same way that we try to increase their understanding of children.

Sociocultural Supplies
Preventive action in regard to ensuring the sociocultural

supplies of the aged population includes modifying retirement laws and regulations so that people who retain their
capacities are not forced to retire suddenly and prema-
turely and may be offered part-time or lighter work opportunities as their powers diminish. Old age assistance and
retirement pensions should take up the slack in income
as earning capacity is reduced by age. These regulations
should not penalize a person for working. In certain cases,
at present, the lowered earning capacity of older people
means that their income may be less if they work than
if they were entirely unemployed and drawing full welfare
assistance.

Social isolation is a potent factor in promoting mental
disorders in the aged. A preventive program should foster
the provision of social and recreational facilities and
should be administered so that the activity and independence of the old people will be stimulated, rather than
encouraging them to become the passive recipients of
care. In preparation for this, health education programs
aimed at the middle-aged population should take the form
of anticipatory guidance, so people face the implications
of old age ahead of time and see this period as one in
which they will be expected and encouraged to remain
interested in the social, political, welfare, and recreational
life of their community, and be productively active in formal work or service, and later in sheltered occupations.

The most obvious example of ensuring the provision of
sociocultural supplies in a program of primary prevention
is that of influencing the educational system. The role of
psychiatrists in offering consultation to educators on curriculum matters and in helping them improve the mental
health atmosphere of the school is well known. A special
example relates to a preventive psychiatry program which
has recently been initiated in a metropolitan slum. In that
area the scholastic levels of many young people who leave

high school are no longer sufficient for the demands of the labor market, because rapid technological advances have lowered the traditional need for unskilled labor. The result has been rising unemployment among young people whose inadequate education has made them occupationally redundant. This has had obvious effects on their psychological well-being; they are frustrated and restless and tend to rebel against the social order which they feel is rejecting them. The neighborhood is reported to have an increased incidence of delinquency, alcoholism, drug addiction, illegitimate pregnancies, abortion, and venereal disease, which would seem logically linked to this situation. Attempts to deal with this problem by traditional casework and remedial psychiatric practices have had a similar effect to bailing out a flooded room with a small bucket while the water continues to pour in from a burst pipe. Instead, a new preventive service has been instituted which attempts to handle the problem at its source. A systematic program of improving the educational offerings of the school system in that neighborhood has been instituted. Extra teachers of high caliber have been hired. Modern educational techniques are being used. At the same time, the level of aspiration of the students and their families is being dramatically raised by involving the whole community in an adult educational campaign. This increases the motivation of the students to stay at school and to study as hard as students in middle-class school districts, with the hope and the confidence that the technologically advanced labor market will be open for them to enter also.

In all these examples the preventive psychiatrist identified a deprivation of physical, psychosocial, or sociocultural supplies in his community and then undertook social action to remedy the defect. He carried out educational campaigns to change the attitudes of professional or lay groups, or he influenced legislators and administrators to modify laws, regulations, and policies. In connection with the latter, it is worth emphasizing that I am not advocating government by psychiatrists. Legislators and administrators will take into consideration many economic, social, and political issues before making their decisions. The mental health issue may to them have a lower priority than these, and the psychiatrist's pleas may therefore fall on deaf ears. Primary prevention, however, demands that the psychiatrist make his voice heard, so that those who govern may at least take into account the basic mental health needs of their population; and so that if they infringe upon these they may do so knowingly, and perhaps accept the responsibility of dealing with the unhappy consequences. For example, the psychiatrist may point out that an urban relocation program is likely to have a mentally unhealthy effect on the aged inhabitants of a condemned area. The economy of the city may nevertheless demand that the slum be torn down and replaced by modern apartment houses. The legislators, who have been warned of the human consequences, may then feel obligated to provide extra social work and home-nursing service to the old people, giving them special help in handling their relocation difficulties. The legislators may also be inclined to solicit the advice of the psychiatrists in planning other measures to cushion the blow, such as making provision for ethnic and extended family groups to be rehoused near each other, and near the places where their old social and recreational agencies have been relocated.

The Significance of Life Crises

Crises are the short periods of psychological upset which occur from time to time as a person wrestles with problems which are temporarily beyond his capacity. If we analyze the life histories of patients suffering from mental disorders we usually find that sudden deteriorations in mental health occurred immediately following such crises. It appears that during the crises significant psychological changes must have occurred. Such findings point to the potential value of studying what takes place during crises in order to find a leverage point for improving the mental health outcome.

The upset of a crisis is caused when the person is confronted by an important life problem from which he cannot escape and which he cannot solve in a short time in his usual way. The source of the problem may be primarily internal and be due to physiological or psychological upheavals associated with development, such as the internal changes of puberty, pregnancy, menopause or old age; or it may be primarily in the environment and be caused by physical or psychosocial changes—the so-called situational crisis. There are three main types of environmental problems which precipitate situational crises: first, the loss of a source of satisfaction of basic needs, such as the death or departure of a loved person, or a loss of bodily integrity, such as a crippling illness or the amputation of a limb; second, the danger of such a loss; and third, a challenge which overtaxes a person's capacities, such as a sudden job promotion for which he is not adequately prepared.

During a crisis the individual's usual pattern of functioning becomes disorganized. He feels upset and emotionally disturbed. He becomes confused and ineffective. He is tense, restless, and irritable and may be anxious, angry, or depressed. He is preoccupied with the problem which precipitated the upset and often by memories of similar problems from the past. He feels frustrated because he is not able to deal with the situation.

The crisis may last for a period of up to 4 to 6 weeks.

By the end of that time, the tension usually abates and the person returns to a steady psychological state; he eventually works out some new way of dealing with the crisis problem through making use of unexpected or untried capacities in himself and through enlisting new sources of help in those around him. He may deal with the problem in a healthy, adaptive way by realistically modifying the environment or by adjusting in a socially acceptable way to the changed situation. On the other hand, he may find some way of evading the issue, by pretending the problem does not exist or denying its importance, or he may resort to irrational mental gymnastics which persuade him that he has solved the problem, even though he has not really faced it. For example, a bereaved person may operate as though the deceased were still alive. He may also end the crisis by developing psychiatric symptoms that preoccupy him or alienate him from the reality world in which the problems exist.

The novel response he develops in dealing with the crisis problem, whether healthy or maladaptive, becomes a new part of his coping and is available thereafter for use when he deals with future problems.

If the solution is a socially acceptable, reality-based adaptive response, he emerges from the crisis with an increased potential for mental health—that is, for dealing realistically with future problems. If it is maladaptive, he emerges with a greater vulnerability to mental disorder, which shows itself either in the near future or after similar responses to subsequent crises has taken him still further along the road of irrationality.

At each successive crisis he will have his chance over again to choose the path towards mental health or else towards mental disorder, but with the dice loaded more and more in one direction or the other by his past choices.

Crises therefore represent mental health turning points or way stations. The balance may come down on one side or the other; there is the opportunity for a healthier development and the danger of a move towards pathology.

During the period of the struggle the person in crisis is usually not alone. He will be helped or hindered in finding a healthy outcome by his family and friends, and by the people in his community to whom he may turn for help and guidance, such as doctors, lawyers, teachers, clergymen, and social workers. These people may influence him in one direction or another.

Two other facts about crisis are important for preventive psychiatry: A person in crisis feels a greater need for help than when he is in his usual psychological state. He reaches out for help, and the signs of his crisis upset usually stimulate the people around to respond to his request.

The second phenomenon is that during crisis a person *is more easily influenced* than at other times. He is in unstable equilibrium like a person standing on one leg—a slight push tips his balance to one side or the other. The same push when he is in equilibrium, standing on both legs, would have little effect.

Crisis therefore represents a leverage point. Not only is it a way station, but the person can be more easily influenced at such a time to choose a mentally healthy path. He is both willing and susceptible to being influenced by minimal interventions.

This means that a small amount of helping effort will produce a much bigger effect if focused on people at crisis times than if applied to people in stable equilibrium. Here then is an opportunity to maximize the potential of our scarce mental health specialists.

Preventive Services in Relation to Crisis

These ideas about crisis have been derived from a series of researches carried out over the past fifteen years on such examples as the crisis of bereavement, the reactions of parents to the birth of a premature or congenitally deformed baby, the crises of surgical patients, or of people adjusting to a diagnosis of tuberculosis. We have lately also studied the crises experienced by Peace Corps Volunteers exposed to unexpected cultural problems in their overseas assignments, and by engaged and newly married couples in dealing with the ordinary upsets of early married life.

Based on the findings of such studies, we have developed the following methods of preventive psychiatry.

Reducing the Severity of Crises in a Community

It is not feasible to prevent crises altogether. Temporarily insurmountable problems are an inevitable aspect of everyone's life. There will always be unexpected and unwelcome situations to be faced such as illness, death, accidents, and operations. Normal development implies novelty and change. Even if it were possible to obviate all stress and challenge, we would not wish to do so because the successful mastery of such problems provides the opportunity for personality growth and enrichment.

It does appear, however, that if the stresses can be kept within bounds, the crisis upsets will be less intense and there will be a better chance of healthy adaptive responses.

The preventive psychiatrist will therefore monitor the living conditions of his community in order to identify the hazardous circumstances which will precipitate crisis in significant numbers of the population. He will then seek to modify these circumstances on a community-wide scale so that their crisis-inducing impact is reduced.

For instance, the death of a loved one provokes crisis

in almost everyone. In a community with well-established religious traditions, the preventive psychiatrist might not feel called upon to intervene because the attenuation of this crisis would have been ensured by such religious mourning practices as the wake, the funeral ceremony, and the condolence calls of friends and clergyman, all of which have been developed and ritualized over the centuries as effective ways of softening the blow and supporting the bereaved in accepting the inevitability of his loss.

The community may, however, contain subpopulations at special risk who do not belong to stable religious groups which safeguard their interests in this way. Such people may be served by undertakers whose commercial interests focus on arranging funerals which are as quick and free of fuss as possible. The absence of religious ritual which actively involves the mourner in the physical act of burying the dead, although it saves both the undertaker and the bereaved time and effort, may add significantly to the difficulty of the psychological tasks of mourning. These demand the active giving up of the link with the deceased by "psychologically burying" him. The preventive psychiatrist would therefore seek to involve the appropriate community authorities in controlling the practices of undertakers so that the rights of persons who are not members of recognized religious sects are safeguarded.

The hazards of mourning would also be reduced if the bereaved person were freed for a period from the demands of his job so that he could devote his energies to the psychological work of adjusting to his loss—to do what some people have called his "grief work." Many religions prescribe such a period of retirement, like the Jewish "shivah" or seven days of deep mourning. The possibility is suggested that public education and the modification of policy in industry might lead to the widespread adoption of the practice of offering "mourning leave" with pay, analogous to "sick leave."

Services to Foster Healthy Crisis-Coping

The outcome of a crisis is modified by the help or hindrance which the individual receives from family and friends, and from people of influence in the community, while he is trying to work out a pattern of adjustment and adaptation to the upsetting circumstances. The preventive psychiatrist and his mental health specialist colleagues are part of this potentially helpful influence network. They may personally help people in crisis, but this number is not likely to be very large. Their major impact must come from indirect action. This may take the following paths.

Ensuring Provision of Professional Help During Crisis

In order for professional workers to help a person in crisis, it is necessary for them to understand the nature of crisis reactions and to have the skill to influence him to adopt a healthy approach to his crisis tasks. They must also be available to offer this help during the relatively short periods of crisis disequilibrium when his choices of coping pattern are being made. We can rely on the increased desire for help during crisis to impel the person to ask for assistance; but unless he can gain access to the helper during the crisis period itself—a period no more than a few weeks in duration—he will have to cope unaided with his tasks.

This situation presents no problem in many types of crisis, because the predicament itself is so clearly a life emergency that immediate contact with a community agency or care-giving professional is mandatory, as with a surgical emergency, a road accident, or a death in the family. In many other instances, however, the predicament, apart from the psychological crisis, is not an obvious emergency, as in the crises of adolescence, early marriage, change of job, or the loss of a loved one by disillusionment or relocation. In these cases the individual in crisis must reach out for help from a health, welfare, education, or religious agency. Unfortunately many of these agencies are not at all geared to handling new cases quickly. They have long waiting lists, and they operate on the assumption that they deal mainly with chronic cases in which the time factor is significant only in regard to the duration of treatment, and not in regard to its immediate availability. Such agencies usually conceive of an emergency case as one of dramatic severity. Only such cases are likely to be given priority on their waiting lists. Crisis upsets are evanescent and minor in intensity, and therefore would not naturally be considered urgent.

Preventive psychiatrists must therefore seek to influence agency administrators to change their policies so that their doors should be readily opened on demand to persons in crisis, and so that administrative practices may be modified to provide staff for immediate help. Re-education of staff must also be involved, because the new ways of working will confront them with many novel problems, which in turn demand the development of new procedures.

The preventive psychiatrist must also survey the commonly occurring crises in his community and see whether any major categories fall outside the sphere of current agency operations. If so, he must try and influence the community legislative and planning bodies either to assign new jurisdictions to old agencies or to establish new agencies to cover areas of unmet need. One example is the absence of adequate homemaker services in many communities. Their provision to ensure that families facing the crisis produced by the temporary absence of mothers may be kept together in their homes, instead of being split up, must be a major goal of preventive psychiatry. In many communities no agencies are available to assist widows or parents who are divorced. The Cruse Clubs in England and Parents Without Partners in this country have grown up in recent years to deal with these problems, and their development should clearly be fostered by preventive psychiatrists. In some communities, especially in rural areas, many traditional family and child-welfare agencies are missing; their provision must be a major goal of those involved in the primary prevention of mental disorder.

Education of Caregivers

The caregiving professionals—the doctors, nurses, clergymen, teachers, and lawyers—are the major source of community aid to people in crisis. If we wish to ensure that these caregivers pay special attention to the mental health implications of the crisis, and act skillfully to influence the upset person and his family to cope in a healthy manner; they must be educated in regard to the significance for subsequent mental health of coping patterns in crisis; they must learn enough about various crises to know what specific tasks are involved in each, and what is the range of healthy and unhealthy patterns of accomplishing them, in order that they may be able to identify those individuals who are proceeding on a maladaptive course. They must also learn how to influence such persons to modify their ways of coping in a healthy direction. For instance, in the crisis of premature birth, doctors and nurses should be aware that the pattern of the mother's initial adjustment to the situation may have a significant effect on her subsequent relationship to and care of her child. They should learn to identify mothers who are coping poorly; like the mother who seems overly cheerful and unconcerned about the situation; who shows little curiosity about her baby's progress and about the meaning of prematurity; who visits him infrequently in the premature nursery; and who does not seek help from family members, friends, and professionals in dealing with the problems involved, which on the whole she tends to evade or deny. Those helping such a mother cope more adequately, can influence her to pay more attention to some of the problems and can support her in admitting to consciousness and mastering the feelings of anxiety, frustration, and deprivation which are then likely to emerge. Her knowledge of prematurity and its problems can be enlarged by discussion of different aspects of the crisis. She can be encouraged to visit her baby regularly and to learn how to understand and predict his progress by observing his behavior and by getting relevant information from the nurses. She can be assisted to enlist the support of other people in handling the problems which emerge; and she can be helped to make appropriate contacts with clergymen, public health nurses, and physicians, as indicated.

Such results can be achieved if preventive psychiatrists study the expectable phenomena of the common crises in their community, either personally or from the research literature, and then communicate this knowledge to the other caregivers by taking part in their preprofessional education or by participating in on-the-job training in postgraduate seminars for teachers, clergymen, or general practitioners.

Mental Health Consultation

However well educated the community caregivers are in regard to crisis work, it is inevitable that they will encounter unexpected difficulties as they engage in such preventive activities. This is more likely because of the emotionally "hot" nature of a crisis which is apt to interfere with their professional distance and objective judgment. In order to consolidate a program of preventive work by caregivers it is therefore important to provide them with opportunities for consulting a mental health specialist whenever they encounter a work situation which they find confusing. Over the last ten years methods of consultation have been developed for use by mental health specialists in dealing with this issue. For instance, the Laboratory of Community Psychiatry in Boston, which this author directs at Harvard Medical School, sends a mental health specialist for a couple of hours every week into each of the twenty health stations out of which the public health nurses of the Health Department and the Visiting Nurse Association operate. Nurses who are having difficulties dealing with crises or other psychologically complicated issues in their patients are free to ask for consultation. This system provides an opportunity for the public health nurses to clarify the complexities of their cases, which enables them and their supervisors to work out improved ways of helping their patients deal with their current life difficulties. In other areas of Massachusetts and also in California, similar consultation programs are available in schools and in other community agencies.

Education of Informal Caregivers

People in crisis often turn for help not to the professional caregivers but to people who live or work near them. They have learned to know and respect these people as counselors even though they have no official professional helping status. Such informal caregivers include wise neighbors, men who work in corner drugstores, bartend-

ers, hairdressers, industrial foremen, and the like. They
are chosen by people as confidants because of special personality gifts—a capacity for empathy and understanding,
and an interest in their fellow men. They are often complicated people with personal problems of their own, who
have been sensitized by these to the sufferings of others.

These informal caregivers exert a significant influence
on the mental health of the population, and pose a major
problem for preventive psychiatry. How can we make
contact with them, and how can we educate them so that
they give wise counsel to those in crisis who seek them
out? They have no formal training, and we have no hand
in selecting them.

The only way of reaching them seems to be through
the mass media. One example of what can be done was
shown in a 1962 article written by the journalist Vivian
Cadden in the monthly magazine, *Redbook*. It is entitled
"Crisis in the Family," and is addressed to those to whom
people in crisis turn for help. It discusses the implications
of crisis-coping for mental health, and then describes the
results of studies which clarify the healthy and unhealthy
patterns of dealing with crisis problems. It points out that
when a person is in crisis he is not likely to make personal
use of such knowledge because he will be psychologically
confused and upset. His family and friends, or others to
whom he turns for help, may not be emotionally involved
to the extent that their judgment is distorted, and so they
will be in a position to help him take a balanced view
of his situation. The article makes it clear that there are
no set prescriptions for dealing adaptively with crisis, but
it concludes with a series of guidelines or basic principles
which may be useful in the helping process.

This article has been received with much interest. It
has been reprinted in other periodicals with mass circula-
tions, such as the *Catholic Digest*, and it has been repub-

lished as a pamphlet which has been distributed widely in industrial settings. It points to the possibility of an educational campaign which can be beamed to informal caregivers, not only through the written word but also via radio and television.

Personal Preparation for Healthy Crisis-Coping Through Education

Another approach which seeks a population-wide effect is to modify the content and methods of the education of children and youth so that general skills are acquired for dealing adequately with unexpected and temporarily insoluble problems.

One way of achieving this has been developed by Dr. Ojemann of Iowa (1962). He has criticized the usual type of education in this country as leading to what he calls "surface thinking," whereby behavior in any situation is rather simply and automatically determined as a reaction to the overt manifestations of the problem. In place of this he advocates a "causal approach" in which the person always seeks to uncover the causes of the observed manifestations and then systematically works out a plan of action to deal with the most crucial of these causes. He has rewritten school textbooks and he has trained teachers in methods of teaching this causal thinking as an integral part of the normal school curriculum. He has evaluated the results of his method by comparing children taught along his lines with similar children from traditional classes, and has demonstrated that children taught the "causal approach" are better at solving novel problems. They have an increased capacity to persevere in the face of ambiguity, and they have an increased tolerance of frustration. These are precisely the attributes which make for an improved capacity to deal adaptively with crisis.

Another approach is that of Kurt Hahn and the Outward Bound movement in Britain (1957), which has been one of the sources of our own Peace Corps. This takes the form of a character-building type of experiential education for adolescents and young adults. The students are exposed to situations of natural hazard, such as climbing mountains or ocean sailing—or in the Peace Corps, physical deprivation and cultural conflict. The stress is graduated so as to be just beyond the usual capacity of the student. He experiences a crisis upset, and he is then provided with adult support and guidance in working his way through to a healthy adaptation. This leads to a strengthening and maturing of his personality, with increased independence and awareness of his own capacities, and improved skills in making use of the help to be derived from others.

These two successful approaches point to the possibility of modifying our educational system on a widespread basis so as to improve the potential of students to master life crises. It is a field in which collaboration of preventive psychiatrists with educators may yield important results in the future.

Anticipatory Guidance

A recent study by Janis of Yale (1958) has shown that if one observes patients awaiting operation in a surgical ward, it is possible to predict which of them will have the least troublesome postoperative psychological adjustment. The ones who are moderately worried about the operation and ask a lot of questions about the pain and discomfort ahead do much better afterwards than those who seem unusually cheerful and express unconcern about the impending stress. The study also demonstrates that if a person facing a crisis finds out ahead of time what is in store for him and begins to worry about it, he will be better prepared psychologically to handle the strain when the difficulties begin in reality. Janis recommends, on the basis of his research, that patients awaiting operation should be given a sort of "emotional inoculation," whereby they are told in some detail what is likely to happen so that they have a chance to begin to wrestle with the emotional problems and achieve some mastery in advance.

A similar approach has been used for some years in public health, especially in preparing pregnant women for the stress of childbirth and in preparing mothers for dealing with expectable problems in the growth and development of their children. Public health workers have coined the term anticipatory guidance for this type of preventive activity.

In the Peace Corps we have made effective use of anticipatory guidance techniques in preparing volunteers to face the rigors and challenges of overseas service. Some of this preparation has been done by psychiatrists as a special mental health sequence in Peace Corps training programs. A pamphlet, *Adjusting Overseas*, is read by every trainee. It describes the stresses such as loneliness, strange living conditions, different value systems, boredom, and lack of obvious signs of accomplishment which volunteers must expect overseas, and lets them know they will probably become depressed, anxious, angry, and confused when exposed to these conditions. The psychiatrist then meets with the trainees in a series of small group discussions and helps them evoke the negative feelings they are likely to have as they go through these difficulties. They then begin to learn how to master these feelings by personal adjustments and also by enlisting the emotional support of each other and of the Peace Corps staff.

The Role of the Mental Health Specialist in Relation to Crisis

In addition to his main task of helping the other community caregivers improve their services to people in crisis and offering consultation to community leaders in order to reduce the intensity of crisis-provoking situations, the mental health specialist should spend part of his time in dealing directly with crisis upsets. He is not likely to affect many people this way, but he can use this experience to learn more about the phenomena of crisis which he can incorporate in his educational and consulting work. He can also deal with the more difficult cases which resist the efforts of the other caregivers.

Direct preventive intervention by the specialist should be focused not only on the person in crisis but also on the network of people who are meaningful in his life—his family and friends, and the professionals who care for him. Because of the need for speed in order to capitalize on the increased susceptibility to influence during the crisis, the specialist should do most of this work, not in his own clinic or hospital to which people come by referral, but in community situations where people in crisis normally congregate. He should visit surgical wards, prenatal clinics, well-baby clinics, churches, and schools. There he should build up collaborative relationships with the other professionals so that they may call upon him to see their clients who are currently in crisis. In some of these cases the specialist will intervene himself, and in others he will suggest that the other professionals should do the work with his educational and consultative guidance.

References

Bowlby, J. *Maternal care and mental health.* Geneva: World Health Organization, 1952.

Cadden, V. Crisis in the family. *Redbook*, January, 1962.

Caplan, G. *Principles of preventive psychiatry.* New York: Basic Books, 1964.

Caplan, G. and Cadden, V. *Adjusting overseas: A message to each Peace Corps trainee.* Washington, D.C.: The Peace Corps, 1967.

James, D. (Ed.). *Outward bound.* London: Routledge and Kegan Paul, 1957.

Janis, I. *Psychological stress.* New York: Wiley, 1958.

Joint Commission on Mental Illness and Health. *Action for mental health.* New York: Basic Books, 1961.

Kennedy, J. F. Message from the President of the United States relative to mental illness and mental retardation. Document 58, 88th Congress, First Session, House of Representatives, February 5, 1963.

Ojemann, R. H. Investigations on the effects of teaching an understanding and appreciation of behavior dynamics. In Caplan, G. (Ed.), *Prevention of mental disorders in children, Initial explorations.* New York: Basic Books, 1961.

Ryan, W. *Report of the Boston mental health survey to the advisory and steering committees.* Cosponsored by Massachusetts Association for Mental Health, Massachusetts Department of Mental Health (Division of Mental Hygiene), and the United Community Services of Metropolitan Boston, 1962.

United States Department of Health, Education, and Welfare. Regulations: Community Mental Health Centers Act 1963. UN *Federal Register*, May 6, 1964.

9

The Nurse's Role in Changing Health Services*

Bill 65, enacted by the National Assembly of Quebec on December 24, 1971, establishes as the main goals of its reorganization of health and social services in the Province to do the following:

Improve the state of the health of the population, the state of the social environment in which they live and the social conditions of individuals, families and groups; . . . make accessible to every person, continuously and throughout his lifetime, the complete range of health services and social services, including prevention and rehabilitation, to meet the needs of individuals, families and groups from a physical, mental and social standpoint; . . .

Every person has the right to receive adequate, continuous and personal health services and social services. . . .

Health services and social services must be granted without discrimination or preference based on the race, colour, sex, religion, language, national extrac-

*A lecture delivered at 77th Reunion of Royal Victorial Hospital Nurses Alumnae Association, McGill University, Montreal, May 8, 1972.

tion, social origin, customs or political convictions of the person applying for them or of the members of his family.

These are inspiring words. They are in line with sentiments recently expressed by other governments in progressive countries throughout the world. However, nobody so far has succeeded in achieving these ambitious goals, although many legislators, administrators, health and welfare researchers and practitioners have been grappling with the complicated issues involved. In this article I will present my personal views about the basic principles of reorganizing health and welfare services to achieve these goals. My ideas are derived from my analysis of the efforts of gifted workers in this field, particularly the pioneers of comprehensive community mental health programs in the United States, who have been actively engaged in developing population-oriented services since the passage of our federal Community Mental Health Centers Act in 1963.

Principles of a Population-Oriented Health and Welfare Service Delivery System

Focus on Satisfying Needs of Individuals in their Families

Planning must start with the individual patient or client; our services must be developed to satisfy his needs rather than, as in the past, building hospitals, clinics, and other institutions and then recruiting customers who have often been forced into procrustean beds to satisfy the needs of the organization.

Important issues include the following:

The presenting patient must be seen as an integral part

of his family. His discomfort or disability may often be one sign of a family disequilibrium due to strain in the physical, psychosocial, sociocultural, and socioeconomic aspects of the lives of its members. The index case comes to the attention of health and welfare workers, but other family members may be in equal or greater need of help in their own right, apart from whatever contribution they may be making to the onset or perpetuation of trouble in the presenting patient. Service must deal with the entire family in order to be effective.

People in difficulty usually have many different troubles. The old medical tradition of parsimony in differential diagnosis, which enjoins the physician to search for a single lesion or illness in explaining all his patient's signs and symptoms, can no longer be regarded as an adequate guide. If we open our eyes to the total existential situation of our patients we will usually see that they are responding physically, mentally, spiritually, socially, and occupationally, in a complicated way, to a complex of difficulties spread over their individual and family history in adjusting to a changing environment. The single illness of the medical diagnostician may be only one of the aspects of the current predicament. Occasionally, as in an acute appendicitis, it may be the most urgent and demand a relatively simple intervention; but even in such a case we may miss factors that are crucial to the present and future well-being of the patient and his family if we restrict our view to McBurney's Point and its physical surroundings.

Since people in trouble have a variety of problems it is hard for them to pre-categorize themselves and decide which is the "presenting complaint" and therefore to which caregiver they should go for help: a physician, a nurse, a social worker, a clergyman, an educator, a lawyer, or a vocational counsellor. All may be relevant, and their salience may change over time.

The needs of an individual and his family are so varied that our services must be manned by very broadly skilled generalists or we must provide a great number of different specialists. In the latter case we must arrange for smooth and rapid contact between patient and relevant specialists, and since any patient is likely to have many special needs at any point in time this presents logistic problems of great difficulty.

Focus Also on the Entire Population

Collectively, we accept responsibility for providing service to all members of the population with current health and welfare needs and for reducing their future needs, both to ensure their well-being and to save ourselves the effort of eventual diagnostic and remedial intervention. This is a tall order, since the potential demand for service is so vast. The total demand will always be greater than we can ever satisfy with our limited economic and professional manpower resources. We must, therefore, plan carefully how to deploy these resources so as to maximize our service delivery and to focus it on those in greatest need. We must also seek ways of augmenting our professional and institutional services by fostering the supportive forces within the population itself. The following issues are relevant:

Pooling Manpower

We must utilize the resources of all caregivers in the community and not limit ourselves to the reorganization of health and welfare services. This means that we must find ways of harnessing the efforts of all potentially relevant professionals and agencies to serve the needs of particular individuals and families. These will include all public and private workers in such fields as health, welfare, education, vocational, religious, recreational, legal, law enforceent, and corrections. Our aim should rarely be the addition of new professionals and institutions because of our shortage of money and manpower, but the reorganization of institutional policies and practices and the concomitant re-education of staffs to take on new roles. The crucial challenge will be to alter the boundaries of agency and professional domains so that their efforts can be integrated in new ways to satisfy the needs of individuals and groups.

Conserving Manpower

We must continually seek methods of conserving professional manpower. One way of accomplishing this is to organize our programs in echelons, like the armed services. At the local level we should work mainly through generalists who should be responsible for triage and for dealing with as many problems as possible at that level. In view of the heterogeneity of problems and their spread over the boundaries of many traditional professional domains, this involves working out methods for convening other professionals and involving them in collaboration on cases. Problems demanding more specialized skills must be temporarily referred to regional and central facilities for handling by specialists, but the local practitioners must retain case responsibility because they must maintain contact with the families and eventually deal with rehabilitation of the patients.

Priorities

An important way of coping with scarcity of resources is to develop a population priority system. The goal is to focus effort on those cases of highest need where remedy is feasible. This is far from simple, especially in a large and heterogeneous population which is continually changing so the needs of individuals and groups are altering differentially over time in response to modifications in them and in their environments. An essential basis for our program must therefore be a mechanism for monitoring the population in order to keep cumulative records of changes in harmful environmental factors and in the characteristics of sub-populations to identify the people who are currently in greatest trouble or exposed to circumstances that involve the greatest risk of physical, mental, or social disorder. These risk or trouble registers will help us to define which groups are in most need at any particular time, and alert us to provide them with appropriate preventive or remedial and rehabilitative services. The registers will also pinpoint harmful environmental situations which demand community action for their amelioration. Unless such monitoring is undertaken as a specific task by a part of the service organization that is responsible for planning and stimulating remedial action, it is likely that little will be done in this field except when a chance crisis of dramatic proportions attracts public attention. The anti-poverty movement in the United States during the past few years has also drawn to our attention that the poor and deprived groups in the population, as well as those who are the object of racial, religious, or ethnic discrimination, are the sub-populations who are likely to be at highest risk and yet to be most often not visible to middle class professionals and their agencies, unless we systematically scan the entire community and then evaluate relative priorities in delivering available services.

The Ecological Systems Model

Planners of comprehensive community services have recently developed a potent conceptual model to guide their efforts. It is usually called the ecological systems model. This model envisages a kind of equation. On one side are the sub-populations in need or at risk, consisting of families in disequilibrium because of psychobiosocial or socioeconomic stress and manifesting in their individual members a variety of symptoms of disorder such as physical or psychiatric illness, social or occupational disability, educational, religious, or legal problems. On the other side of the equation are the caregiving professionals and agencies of the community. The model calls for the latter to be convened into a cohesive caregiving network that should articulate with the needs of the family members and develop a sensible plan to satisfy them by collaborative action. The family problem may be identified by one or more of the caregivers because a family member will come to his attention through manifesting a sign of strain relevant to his profession. For instance, the father may come to the notice of the police because of being drunk and disorderly, the mother may be referred to a hospital because of high blood pressure, a son may be identified as a problem in school because of academic underachievement, a teenage daughter may be referred to a social agency because of a pregnancy out of wedlock. According to the ecological systems model, whichever professional identifies the family problem should scan the family as a whole and then convene all the other relevant caregivers who are active or who should be active on the case. The group of caregivers then builds up a comprehensive view of the family stresses, strains, and capacities by each worker contributing his own perception. This allows the group to develop a joint remedial plan to swing the disequilibrium over in a healthy direction, hopefully by discovering some leverage points that were not visible to each because of his partial view of the situation. In our previous case example this turned out to be arranging English lessons and vocational training for the father of the immigrant family in New York so that he could get a job commensurate with his abilities, regain his status as a respectable head of the family, and exercise leadership to raise the morale of the family and control its members.

Prevention

Even in the best of all possible worlds the above improvements in efficiency, logistics, and collaboration of caregiving professionals and their rational deployment to deal with those in greatest need who can benefit from service, although a great improvement over our present situation, will still not solve more than a fraction of the health and welfare needs of the population. These professional measures must be complemented by an active campaign of prevention of disorder through reducing harmful environmental factors and increasing the capacity of individuals, families, and neighborhood groups to master environmental stresses and challenges, largely by fostering the helpful activity of nonprofessionals, and particularly person-to-person self-help support systems in the community. Organizations such as Alcoholics Anonymous, Synanon, the La Leche League, Widow-to-Widow programs, Parents Without Partners, Ileostomy and Mastectomy Associations, as well as peer counselling in high schools and colleges and informal mutual help by neighbors at crisis times organized by religious groups or as a spontaneous part of neighborhood tradition—all these and many more are beginning to be recognized as an essential ingredient in comprehensive community health and welfare programs. Of particular importance is the fact that when a nonprofessional helps a person in need, both benefit from the process. We professionals must appreciate the significance of nonprofessional efforts and we must learn how to support them. We must develop sufficient respect for our own contributions and sufficient personal and group security not to attack or defensively

belittle the nonprofessionals as though they were competing with professionals. They complement the professionals; they cannot replace them.

In recent years we have come to realize that in the
fields of mental health and welfare, and in many aspects
of physical health and illness, it is important not to
remove a sufferer from his natural milieu either literally
or by labelling him as defective or deviant. By keeping
him inside his social group and in his familiar surroundings, he is more likely to struggle actively to master the
stress and to mobilize the support of his social network;
if he is removed or alienated, he is likely to regress to
a more passive and weak condition. Only if his active
struggle in his natural surroundings does not lead to mastery in a reasonable time should he be brought into the
professional helping system, and then only for a minimum
period, while maintaining as much as possible his links
with family, neighbors, and friends whose supports and
reality-based expectations will be so important in the
eventual rehabilitation process.

This means that we should try hard to organize all our
professional institutions to be as open as possible to their
surrounding community. We should actively involve local
citizens in management of the institutions and we should
recruit volunteers to come in and help with our work.
This is not only an excellent source of extra hands to ease
our professional manpower shortage, but it maintains
open lines of communication across institution boundaries
and helps to prevent our patients from becoming alienated
from their home environments.

Focus on Programs for Bounded Populations
It is important that we should deal with circumscribed
populations, either those who live within certain geographic boundaries called "catchment areas" in the 1963

Community Mental Health Centers Act, or those who are members of a particular organization. In either case we accept responsibility for the care of the total population, the sick, the well, and those who are currently healthy but may eventually become ill. Only by working within such outside boundaries can we succeed in mapping the internal boundaries of the sub-populations with differential characteristics and living conditions that influence their chances of becoming ill, and in determining the epidemiological rates of incidence and prevalence of different health and social disorders, as well as identifying the caregiving professionals and agencies with whom we must collaborate in our program. Eventually we will be called upon to evaluate the results of our efforts, and unless we focus on a circumscribed population we will not be able to document changes in the rates of disorder that we may ascribe to our interventions.

Allotment of Service Responsibilities and Accountability for Population Units

This is probably the crucial issue in organizing our services. The population must be divided up into units of appropriate size, each of which is allotted to a particular group of workers. The work group is given a share of our resources and undertakes responsibility for the comprehensive care of its segment of the population. It is held accountable for the fulfilment of its obligations, as judged by regular evaluations of its operations and its achievements.

The size and composition of the work group depends on the size and characteristics of the population segment allotted to it, and on whether the group works in a front-line echelon operating comprehensively and in a generalized fashion or in a middle or rear echelon with more specialized assignments. Front-line echelon groups usually deal with relatively small population segments of 4-10,000, and if the living conditions are poor and the disorder rate high, even these segments may need to be subdivided among smaller work teams. The important point is that each team should be able to handle all the expectable problems of its population segment for which it accepts responsibility and for which it is held accountable.

Responsibility must be linked with authority; this system can only work if there is maximum decentralization of decision making. Each team is empowered to make whatever decisions are relevant to its own echelon of operations.

Because of the small size of the population segment for which it is responsible, the work team can get to know its potential clients well and can effectively monitor their living conditions. It can also get to know and build good relationships with the other caregiving professionals and agencies upon whom it can call for collaboration in fulfilling its responsibilities. The professional work group can also identify and help to organize the nonprofessional caregivers of that locality.

Experience in many places has shown that if a team of health and welfare professionals is allotted total responsibility for comprehensive coverage of the needs of a small population, it will be forced to innovate a whole range of new techniques of preventive intervention and short term remedies in order to keep abreast of the flow of cases seeking attention. Like the proverbial Chinese physicians they will be rewarded for keeping people healthy and tranquil, rather than for treating them when they are sick, because every failure in prevention will add to their inescapable work burdens. Experience also has taught us that professionals, being human, often attempt to evade their responsibilities in such a system by declining to accept certain cases that they deem undesirable because they are bothersome, unduly time-consuming, or uninteresting. They may do this by overt or covert rejection or by selective inattention. They may accomplish the same goal by a short triage interview followed by referral to some other agency, namely by separating sheep from goats and dumping the undesirables.

A cornerstone principle of our system must therefore be to block these defensive evasions of responsibility. This may be done by prohibiting the decline or export of cases by health and welfare professions in public services. This is in direct opposition to Canada's Item 3, Section 6 of Bill 65 which states that "nothing in this act shall restrict . . . the freedom of . . . a professional to . . . refuse to treat . . ." a resident of the Province of Quebec who "wishes to receive health services or social services. . . ." I fear that this statement may render impossible the achievement of the basic goals of Bill 65.

Of course, professionals in the private sector of our democratic society are perfectly entitled to pick and choose their cases according to their own criteria of age, sex, wealth, beauty, and diagnosis, subject only to the ethical strictures of their professional guilds. Since we need to harness the efforts of as many of the private practitioners as possible in order to achieve coverage of the total population, we deal with this by the equally acceptable free-enterprise strategem of offering them contracts that remunerate them appropriately, but which also bind them to accept every case they receive from the public sector. They retain their freedom to sign or not to sign the contract, but once they have signed, its terms prohibit decline or export and they, like the professionals in the public sector, are held accountable by evaluation of their performance and achievements.

This approach may seem authoritarian and rough on the professionals, but necessity is indeed a hard taskmaster,

and if we are to achieve our goals we must mobilize maximum effort. We must not sacrifice the rights of any
member of the community for his fair share of health and
welfare service to the prejudice or arbitrary preference
of a publicly supported professional.

This approach may be appropriate on moral grounds,
but can it succeed in practice? Our experience in many
places has taught us that it can. What we demand from
the professional is that he should accept every client who
asks him for help and deal with him to the best of his
ability and within the limits of his resources. We do not
stipulate how the worker should accomplish this—it is a
matter for his professional judgment. He will clearly not
have the time or resources to treat every case from
beginning to end on his own. On the contrary, the realis-
tic constraints of this situation will force the professional
to call in as many other community workers and agencies
as possible to help him handle his case load and prevent
him from being swamped. The following organizational
strategems have proved helpful in this connection.

Ensuring Continuity of Care by Means of Agency Consortiums

In many places, community health and welfare agencies
of different types have banded together into consortiums
or combines by negotiating mutually binding legal contracts with each other. These contracts guarantee free
movement of clients among agencies; that is, the client
of one agency must be accepted without delay by all other
agencies in the consortium. The contracts also guarantee
free movement of information about a client. Agencies are
entitled to keep their own private specialized records, but
the fundamental case information must be shared on
request with workers in all other agencies, and is covered
by the overall confidentiality rules of the consortium. In

some places the contracts also provide mechanisms for free movement or sharing of staff, for instance intake into the network may be arranged on a roster basis by representatives of each agency in rotation. A professional who is a specialist in his home agency may work as a generalist in another agency; he may treat cases directly in his own agency and work as a specialist consultant to generalist staff in another agency.

One Door Entry into the System

A basic principle in many comprehensive programs is that people in need of service are not expected to pre-categorize themselves and decide to which of several alternative specialized agencies they should apply for help. They all come to a single address and the responsibility for triage rests entirely with the intake worker who is able to mobilize on their behalf all the generalists and specialists of the service system.

Many front-echelon programs manage this by establishing a network of local multi-service centers, each focused in a single building and staffed by representatives of all the participating public and private community health and welfare agencies. Sharing the same building provides the potential to help clients of all ages who may need help in such fields as health, mental health, clinical and public health nursing, social welfare, law, and vocational guidance and education. If the participating agencies are not bound together by legal consortium agreements, their representatives are at least in a position to build up personal relationships with each other as a basis for informal collaboration in dealing with their allotted population.

The Primary Practitioner Principle

Most programs that operate along these lines emphasize the importance of providing for every client, and if possible for every family, a primary practitioner, a professional who undertakes continuing case responsibility and accountability no matter how many other caregivers may be working on the case. The primary practitioner makes his own generalist or specialist contribution, and in addition appraises the needs of the client and family for help by others, arranges for such service to be obtained, orchestrates the interventions of various professionals and agencies, follows up to monitor the results and the need for changes in the plan, and builds a continuing relationship with the family so that they have somebody they know to whom they can turn in the event of future need, with the assurance of an immediate effective response.

This primary-practitioner function in the health field used to be part of the role of family doctors or general medical practitioners. As increasing medical specialization has all but removed these professionals from the scene in many communities in the United States, a hiatus in health care delivery has begun to be felt. Moreover, a significant part of the population has never had adequate contact with family doctors: the poor, the migrants, and many people in isolated or rural areas. As the fundamental right of every citizen to adequate health and welfare services has become recognized by government, the concept of the primary practitioner has been developed, and his duties have been widened to include not only the traditional health areas, but also the other types of human service. It has also been recognized that since the core activity of a primary practitioner is a generalist scanning and monitoring of needs and harnessing of services, any competent professional can accept this responsibility, and it need not be restricted to physicians.

Replacing Referral of Clients with Collaboration of Professionals

In recent years we have become increasingly disenchanted with the traditional referral system. It is burdensome to clients to be shuttled from agency to agency, being repeatedly appraised to determine if they are appropriate grist for the professional's mill. It is wasteful of scarce professional time and effort to carry out lengthy diagnostic investigations to separate sheep from goats. Moreover, public awareness of need is rising as the fundamental right to service is becoming widely recognized, and community agencies will have to deal with increasing demands. The present situation of a busy agency resenting referral from another institution as a form of "dumping" an unwanted case is therefore likely to be aggravated. The primary practitioner system has suggested a way to deal with this difficulty that is being explored in many service systems, with promising results. A worker who has case responsibility for a client or family and who identifies their need for some specialized service invites the appropriate colleague to help him with his case, rather than trying to get the colleague to take over responsibility for the case, as in the classical referral system. The colleague is more likely to respond positively to this invitation, first because it is a time limited intervention and he knows he can hand back the case for follow-up, and second because he is helping a colleague on whom he himself can call for assistance with one of his own cases when the need arises. This *quid pro quo* approach produces a healthy atmosphere in which both professionals recognize that a collaborative relationship is to their mutual advantage.

Feedback and Evaluation

Apart from the usual motivation of professionals to continually improve the quality of their work and to guide this process by regularly evaluating the effectiveness of their different techniques, workers who are held accountable for the fulfilment of their community responsibilities must develop evaluation instruments to demonstrate objectively what they have achieved.

Over the long haul, evaluation of health and welfare services must focus on documenting changes in the incidence and prevalence of illness and social incapacity in the population. But since many other factors influence these community rates it is difficult to ascribe changes to the preventive or remedial programs, and year-to-year evaluation must usually be restricted to the less objective criteria of consumer satisfaction. This means that population-oriented programs of the kind we have been discussing must make special and continuing efforts to collect feedback information about changes in levels of need for service and about the degree to which people feel that the services are satisfying their needs.

Another relevant issue is that, in contrast with a traditional institution or agency in which the professionals establish their own goals and have no real difficulty in guiding their program to keep on target, a population-oriented service is supposed to be geared to goals that emerge from the felt needs of the potential clientele. Success must therefore be measured not merely by changes in those people who are dealt with by the system, but also by identifying those in the community whose needs were not recognized or satisfied by the caregivers. This is much more complicated. It means that feedback must not be restricted to satisfied clients, but must include unsatisfied clients, and the people in difficulties in the community whose lives were not touched by the program.

Every institution or program has a natural tendency to take on a life of its own and eventually to restrict its intake and modify its operations to satisfy the needs of its staff as much, if not more, than the needs of its potential clients. A number of community health and welfare leaders have lately been trying to minimize this problem by developing mechanisms to increase the sensitivity of program planners and directors to negative feedback that signifies that the program is insensibly drifting off course. Usually the population groups that are liable to be neglected are those who differ in race, class, or culture from the caregivers, and whose cries of pain or frustration are either not loud enough to be heard or are in a language not understood by the community workers.

Methods of ensuring adequate feedback to keep the program on course have included devoting professional effort to regular widespread monitoring of the population; hiring representatives of the different population subgroups, the so-called indigenous nonprofessionals, who have the task of communicating the needs and wishes of their people to the program directors; encouraging lawyers and other professionals to act as advocates for the poor and neglected; paying special attention to dissatisfied clients and to people who were frustrated in their attempts to get help; organizing constituencies of the potential clients as watchdog or pressure committees to monitor the program; and including representatives of the local population on advisory and management councils of the program. The optimal pattern of such feedback mechanisms and ways of bringing the practices of a program back onto the course of sensitivity to the needs of its population will clearly vary from place to place in line with the idiosyncratic character of the local population, but one thing is certain—substantial planning and serious effort must be devoted to this issue if we are to achieve our basic goals.

Roles for Nurses

If plans such as these are ever effectively implemented,

exciting opportunities will become available for nurses. The key roles in the reorganized health and welfare services will be mainly in two areas: first, in system development and management—the central planning and organization to foster maximal decentralization at the echelon levels, and particularly to provide incentives for independent creativity at the local level, using the accountability evaluation mechanisms as a means to promote and reward productive innovation. And second, mastery of the technical problems of implementing the local programs—the primary practitioners, the boundary crossing inside the multiservice centers, the negotiating of consortium agreements, the convening of service networks, and the monitoring of population needs and collection of feedback information. None of these roles has as yet been preempted within traditional professional domains; in various places, similar role functions have been allotted to physicians, nurses, social workers, educators, psychologists, lawyers, and specialists in organization and administration.

The choice of a particular professional group to occupy one of the newly emerging roles will be based on the interaction of a number of factors: the awareness of a specific service need translated into a job description; the recognition that the traditions, training, and experience of that profession provide an adequate basis for acquiring the new skills; the interest of the profession in developing the new role; and the record of pioneering members of that profession in exploring how to develop such skills in comparison with the record of other professions who are competing for the job.

As a friendly observer of nurses over many years, during which I have collaborated with them in various institutional and community settings, I feel this profession has a number of special advantages that will stand it in good stead in competing for the key jobs in reorganized health and welfare programs:

Public Image
The image of nurses among the public is that they can be relied upon to minister with skill and sensitivity to the physical and mental needs of suffering people. The extension of nursing from inpatient to outpatient settings and then to public health work in domiciliary bedside nursing, in prevention, and in health promotion services in the community has widened the field in which nurses are expected to be competent.

History As Generalists
Nurses, particularly public health nurses, have a long history of competence as generalists and therefore are especially qualified to serve at the local echelon of a comprehensive health and welfare service.

Contact
Among all the professionals in the caregiving field nurses have the most regular, frequent, and intimate physical, psychological and social contact with patients and families. Also, nurses are already deployed in large numbers throughout the community, both inside and outside of institutions. They have relatively larger case loads than other professionals. Thus, they already touch the lives of more people in the population than any other profession, and they have a more detailed knowledge of their day-to-day household activities.

Communication Bridges
Because of their range of contact and because nurses have developed a tradition of professional behavior which makes it easy for patients and families of all classes to com-

municate with them, while at the same time their respected position in the health field enables them to communicate fairly easily with physicians and other high status caregivers, nurses are ideally suited to collect feedback information and to act as advocates and communication bridges between the population and the service network.

Professional Skills

In most institution and community settings nurses have always operated as organized groups. They have therefore developed supervisory and administrative skills which have become an integral part of their professional traditions. They have also worked out mechanisms, particularly in public health nursing, to maintain their professional poise and identity when they operate in the open community far from their institutional base.

These characteristics of the nursing profession lead me to the following suggestions about the roles they may succeed in developing within the framework of the reorganized health and welfare system.

A Range of Roles

I believe that nurses should operate at all levels and echelons of the system, as planners, administrators, specialist and generalist practitioners, researchers, and evaluators. Apart from their traditional clinical roles at the bedside and in the clinic and operating room, I do not at present envision any role for the nurses that will be restricted to their profession. On the contrary, I predict that there will be considerable domain overlap, similar to that which is already occurring in many places. Eventually, it may work out in practice that nurses will tend to concentrate on certain parts of the field. This will be based on what pioneers of their profession do over the next few years in innovating the new skills demanded by certain roles; negotiating sanction for their operations among the public and the administrators of programs; feeding the new knowledge back into the reference groups of their profession; building it into their professional traditions; and then standardizing the concepts and practices and handing these on to their professional successors by recruitment, training, and supervision.

Administration Positions

It is hoped that nurses will be appointed to key positions in the administration and planning cadre of the new service, at central, local, and intermediate echelon levels. I expect that their professional tradition in administration and planning will in this regard stand them in good stead.

The Primary Practitioner

The role in the new system that most naturally fits the traditions of the nurse is obviously that of the primary practitioner in a local program. In fact, many district nurses in rural areas have been operating informally along similar lines for many years. In the Soviet Union a network of successful local health centers has been in existence for a long time. Each deals with a population of about 4,000 people and utilizes as its front line generalist a physician who has had six years of training following high school, and who has about the same level of clinical competence as a well-trained nurse in a western country. I believe that a public health nurse with additional clinical and community organizational training, or a clinical nurse with extra public health and community organizational training, could handle with great effectiveness the demands of a primary practitioner job in our projected service.

In a classical multi-service center with rotating intake,

each professional worker in the building would take his turn at receiving cases as a primary practitioner. Here, however, I am referring to a local center whose workers operate in a more differentiated pattern, so that some spend a greater proportion of their time as generalist primary practitioners; this is the role that I feel to be particularly suited to nurses, who are already available in sufficient numbers so that with a little extra training a cadre of appropriate workers could quickly be made available to operate a network of local health and welfare centers.

Boundary Crossing

Another role that should be relatively easy for nurses to move into, on the basis of their existing professional traditions, is that of boundary crossing and negotiation of agreements and relationships among caregivers and their institutions. Public health nurses already do a good deal of this in linking patients with community agencies, and so do hospital nurses in coordinating the movement of patients among the specialized diagnostic and therapeutic department. I have the impression that, in the community, nurses may have a special leverage in convening other professionals to come together to discuss a case in which they each have or should have an interest.

As far back as 1954 I wrote that

"Mobilizing the environment . . . is essentially the province of the nurse. . . . In order to act as the bridge and the mediator between the patient and the specialists, the nurse must be regarded by each as being at the same status level as their own group. She therefore has the difficult task of being 'all things to all men.' "

In that article I discussed the psychological and sociological closeness of the nurse to her patients which made it easy for them to communicate with her. I contrasted this with the difficulty the nurse sometimes has in communicating with physicians and other high status professional specialists. I believe that nurses have made progress in this respect during the past 18 years, but it still remains a problem. On the other hand, the obstacles to what should ideally be horizontal communication among professional peers are not less for the other members of the caregiving network, and nurses at least enjoy the advantage of having many years of experience in consciously grappling with this difficulty.

Monitoring and Feedback

The role in the new service for which the nurse is the most promising contender is that of monitoring the needs for service of individuals and groups and of collecting feedback information to correct deviations of the program from its population-oriented course. Her daily penetration into the homes and lives of all classes in the population, who are united in their common biological vulnerability to illness and intermittent need for nursing care, as well as the easy pooling of her information with that of her nursing colleagues (who cover most of the population) provide a cumulative store of detailed information that no other professional can equal. The only problem in immediately utilizing nurses for this monitoring and feedback role is that they have traditionally been conditioned to neglect this aspect of their functioning, which has not been judged to be important. Because nurses have such large caseloads and because clinical decisions are made by physicians, who usually do not spend much time reading nursing reports, nurses carry much more information in their heads than they include in their records. Moreover, they focus the latter on aspects of getting the job done rather than on the grumblings of patients about dissatisfactions with the health system. If nurses are to play a significant role in collecting and communicating feedback information they will have to enlarge the focus of their interest and to improve their report writing. The decision makers of the program will also have to change their behavior in a complementary manner, and I have no doubt that they will do so if the rewards for such a development are as important an aspect of the new program as I believe they will be.

Implications for Nursing Education

As a population-oriented educator who has been teaching nurses for many years, I cannot finish this chapter without saying a few words about the implications for nursing education of these changes in the health and welfare system and the roles of nurses.

Clearly, responsible participation by nurses in the new service system will extend the traditional boundaries of the profession. The wider the field of independent decision making in the roles I have discussed, the wider and deeper must be the nurse's knowledge. She will need new conceptual maps and a new compass to guide her in unfamiliar territory. She must be prepared to grapple constructively with individual, family, and community crises, and she must learn to think quickly, clearly and cooly during the heat, frustration, and confusion of a crisis period. She must learn new community skills: consultation, community organization, convening of service networks, monitoring noxious environments, and collecting and communicating feedback information. It is therefore appropriate that the site of nursing education should move from the traditional hospital, with its focus on bedside nursing and institutional technology, to the colleges which are oriented more directly to the whole community. The academic setting certainly promises the opportunity of greater faculty sophistication in the scientific and humanistic subjects that provide the basis for professional work in the community. It also brings the education of nurses into closer articulation with that of the other caregiving professionals, so that their future collaboration can be fostered by sharing a generic conceptual vocabulary and way of thinking. But one aspect of this move causes me some concern.

In the traditional hospital nursing school the main teachers were the senior nursing practitioners who had a double claim to high status both as competent professionals and as educators. They not only imparted the theoretical knowledge of nursing, but they also acted as role models in demonstrating professional values, nursing arts, and administrative skills. They played a major part as identification objects in molding the professional self-image of the young nurses. To be sure, some of them were rather narrow in their theoretical vision, but they functioned very well as supervisors and preceptors in helping their students acquire the skills that can only be learned through supervised practicum. Then, there occurred in many hospital nursing schools a much heralded differentiation of the faculty into a semi-autonomous department, and the senior nursing staff split into two groups of educators and practitioners. This probably had advantages in improving the teaching of theory, but it often reduced the opportunity for students to learn from senior practitioners on whom they could model their developing professional identity.

Now there is a more significant move in the same direction. I am concerned lest the opportunity for increased academic sophistication will be gained at the expense of the virtual disappearance of the senior nurse practitioner-role model. On the other hand, if the leaders in nursing education are alert to this danger, they and the administrators of the new health and welfare system may be able to arrange for nurse academicians to spend a significant part of their time in the field of community practice and for senior community nurse practitioners to be also involved actively in nursing education by receiving part-time teaching appointments in the colleges. I hope also that talented practitioners, generalists as well as specialists, at the local level as well as at intermediate and central echelons, will be rewarded in salary and status commensurate with their experience and skill, so that they will represent professionals whom students may wish to emulate and on whom they may thus model their own identities. This is the process which will ensure above all else for the nursing profession the place it deserves in the new health and welfare system.

Reference

Caplan, G. The mental hygiene role of the nurse in maternal and child care. *Nursing Outlook*, January, 1954, Vol. 2, No. 1, pp. 14-19.

10

Conceptual Models in Community Mental Health*

A conceptual model is a pattern for organizing our ideas about a subject so that we can collect meaningful information systematically and plan rational ways of solving significant problems. In the community mental health field, we must develop models which take into account the high incidence and variability of mental disorder; the number and complexity of factors which interrelate in increasing its frequency in the population; and also that in our pluralistic society many people and institutions under a variety of auspices will be engaged in dealing with this vast problem.

The models should tell us which avenues to explore so as to uncover relevant information about particular issues. They should also guide us in developing methods of intervention that maximize the direct impact of our meager specialist resources, and that lead to chain reactions, or ripple effects, in the community which produce a widespread influence through the intermediation of other people and agencies.

This means that we must develop not one but several complementary models, each of which will systematically

*A lecture delivered in 1968 at the Walter Reed Institute of Research, Washington, D.C.

illuminate a particular facet of the multifactorial situation, and which *in toto* will provide us with a comprehensive guide for fact finding and action in the situations we may expect to encounter.

The following are some of the models I regularly use in my everyday operations as a researcher, planner, and practitioner in this field:

Etiological Models

The Nutritional Model

The likelihood of achieving adequate personality development in a population depends on the availability of appropriate opportunities or supplies, in the same way that physical nutrients are needed for adequate bodily development. If a population is deprived of such supplies, especially at certain critical developmental periods of its members, there will be an increased risk of mental disorder.

Mental health supplies can be categorized as physical, psychosocial, and sociocultural. The conditions of life of a population, or of particular subgroups in a population, can be surveyed, and specific deprivations listed: in the physical area, absence of vitamin B in the diet or inadequate protection against lead poisoning; in the psychosocial area, inadequate opportunities for satisfying interpersonal needs because of broken families; in the sociocultural field, poor educational provisions, so that children are not equipped for the expectable job demands in a technologically advanced society, or poor preparation for occupational retirement and poor provisions for maintaining the interest and status of the aged.

This model provides a guide for programs of primary

prevention through identifying and remedying long term damaging factors in the ongoing life situation of population groups.

The Developmental Adjustment or Crisis Model

This is a model with a short term focus on the events and reactions involved at transitional periods of individual development. A person develops through a succession of differentiated phases. Between each phase and the next is a short period of dedifferentiation, upset, or crisis, during which the nature of the succeeding phase is determined, partly by the sum total of what has taken place in that individual's past, and partly by current opportunities and influences.

The focus of the model is upon those current influences during the crisis which can be modified by the intervention of caregivers—educators, helping professionals, administrators, and other people with authority and influence. It points to the opportunity during a crisis of improving the future mental health potential of the individual.

The model is useful in a population-oriented program, because individuals in crisis are more susceptible to influence than during periods of stable equilibrium, so that crisis times are points of leverage. Also, the kind of influence which can tip the balance is essentially that of supportive human relations, and so can be practiced on a widespread scale by interested key people, and usually does not demand the specialized psychological knowledge which would restrict it to use by a relatively small number of highly trained experts.

The crisis model offers a guide to primary prevention by enhancing healthy personality development, to secondary prevention by showing how to use therapeutic workers most efficiently, and to tertiary prevention by identifying the crucial intervention points in preventing and counteracting alienation.

Community Organization and Development Model

This model, which owes much to the research of Alexander and Dorothea Leighton, focuses on the significance for the prevalence of mental disorder of the state of development of a community as a problem-solving organization. If the community has a well-developed pattern of leaders and followers, good communications, an effective control system, and efficient ways of identifying problems and of mobilizing and deploying its resources to deal with them, as well as a value system which accepts the importance of satisfying the human needs of its members, it is likely that the prevalence of mental disorder will be lower than in a similar population and ecological setting which manifests a less developed communal problem-solving structure.

This is a higher-order model than the two previous ones; and it would appear that if a community is well organized and has a humanistic value system, it lowers the risk of mental disorder in its members by ensuring adequate mental health supplies, reducing the impact of crises, and providing services to foster healthy crisis coping in its population.

The model provides a guide for all types of prevention of mental disorder through nonspecific community development, which focuses on the recruitment and training of leaders, improving communication, and helping to work out effective ways of organizing the people so that they learn how to identify salient problems and to mobilize internal and external resources in grappling with them.

Socialization or Effective Role Performance Model

This model emphasizes the significance of complementary role functioning of individuals in a social structure. It focuses on the ways people are recruited and trained for the range of roles needed by society, and on the network of expectations and sanctions which ensure that people behave in ways which keep the social organization in equilibrium.

Within the framework of this model, mental disorder is seen as a condition of deviant functioning in an individual who does not conform to social expectations of appropriate behavior in his roles as a member of his family, work, social, cultural, and religious groups. This deviance is often caused by his inability for a variety of reasons to occupy those roles, and by the ineffectiveness of the usual network of expectations and sanctions in molding his behavior, as well as by the concurrence of his social milieu in supporting his deviant behavior.

The model provides a guide to re-educational or re-socializing ways of bringing the deviant back into line with a socially productive and self-satisfying set of roles in the community. Instead of the disordered person being defined as sick and needing medical treatment in a hospital or clinic administered by a physician, he is seen as a student, apprentice, or trainee, who must be involved in an educational or training program administered and staffed by educators and vocational or industrial training specialists. Issues such as communication, motivation and control by reward and punishment, materials and methods of learning, and individual and group reinforcement become salient, as do ways of organizing training establishments which optimize the fit between current and future individual capacity, and social and occupational demands.

In such settings not only can we recruit the lower level staff from the large available manpower pool in the educational field, as emphasized by Albee, but since the directors are themselves educators, there is an open ladder for career advancement and improved status and salary for all the staff, and therefore opportunity and incentive for professional motivation and consolidation.

It is of interest that many of the first institutions for the rehabilitation of the mentally disturbed in this country in the early nineteenth century moral treatment era were residential educational establishments. They were started by religious educators. Only later did physicians take them over, and for a while they continued to organize them as largely re-educational institutions rather than hospitals.

Models of Practice

Public Health Practice Models

For more than a century, public health workers have been developing models to guide them in preventing and controlling physical illness of populations. A number of their approaches are readily applicable in the mental health field, such as:

Epidemiology. This provides techniques for ascertaining the nature, dimensions, and distribution of the problem in the population. Calculating changes over time in community rates of different disorders in relation to characteristics of subpopulations, and of the social and physical environment, provides guidelines for prevention by uncovering salient etiological factors, and for treatment and rehabilitation by identifying the expectable number and type of cases to be handled.

Planning and Logistics. This model starts from the premise that community resources will always be less than adequate to deal completely with all the current needs. Therefore, it emphasizes the importance of developing a system of priorities in relation to the salience and feasibility of different problems, and then deploying resources in a rational way to deal with those problems in a meaningful order. It also emphasizes evaluation of results and cost accounting, so that the most can be achieved with the available resources.

Catchment Areas. This is a fundamental concept in public health. It refers to a bounded population which can be used as a basis for defining rates of disorder and also as a unit for whose welfare the population-oriented practitioner accepts concern and some measure of responsibility. The responsibility must be sanctioned by some formal community action. Community resources and authority are vested in the practitioner to allow him to do his job, and he is held accountable for his achievement of the allotted goals.

Populations at Risk. An important public health model which helps establish priorities and define goals is that of delimiting subpopulations within the larger community which are particularly demanding of remedial attention or particularly vulnerable and therefore need preventive services. The risk may be related to the native characteristics of the subpopulation such as age, sex, ethnic or social origin, or status as newcomers or transients. It may also be related to current life conditions such as economic or educational deprivation, living in a crowded slum, or being subject to prejudice and racial persecution. Examples of such subpopulations at risk would be children of schizophrenic mothers, who have been shown by studies to have a 40% chance of developing a major mental disorder; aged or infirm people living alone in an area about to be cleared because of urban renewal; young widows; and children whose mothers tried unsuccessfully to abort themselves.

Concepts of Prevention. Public health deals with the problem of controlling the level of disease in a population by focusing its resources in an active preventive manner, rather than passively waiting for difficulties to present themselves for remedy. One public health preventive model that I have found useful is that which divides the field into three levels: Primary prevention, which encompasses measures to reduce incidence—the rate of new cases over a certain time period; secondary prevention, which denotes measures to reduce prevalence—the rate of new and old cases at a point in time; and tertiary prevention, which focuses on lowering the rate of residual defect in the population of former patients.

The Medical Practice or Doctor-Patient Model

In dealing with mental disorders, this model has stood the test of over 150 years of experience. We know its drawbacks, but we also have learned its assets. It defines the mentally disordered individual as a sick person who establishes a contract with a physician to accept him as his patient. The therapeutic relationship is controlled and enriched by centuries of tradition, and it provides for the patient a healer with standardized training and practice, the quality of which is controlled by law, professional ethics, and guild surveillance.

The physician is held personally responsible for safeguarding the welfare of his patient; the latter's individual rights are therefore protected by an effective advocate against possible jeopardy from the organized community system. Moreover, the physician can mobilize the vast network of medical and paramedical resources on behalf of his patient, and can tailor these to the latter's individual needs and rhythm.

Modern psychological medicine views both the etiology and the treatment of a psychiatric patient as multifactorial, and the physician is ideally responsible for orchestrating the manipulation of all types of factors which precipitated and exacerbated the patient's disorder, and the institution of physical, psychosocial, and sociocultural methods of treatment and rehabilitation.

However effective we become in preventing mental disorder, it is likely that there will always be large numbers of acutely and chronically sick individuals in a community who will need attention. The medical practice model provides one important guide to their treatment, and nothing we do in developing other models should be allowed to reduce its being utilized to the fullest possible degree.

The Ecological Systems Model

This model views an individual as an integral part of a succession of open systems, each of which is a subsystem of a larger unit. He may thus be part of a sibling subsystem of a family system, which in turn is a subsystem of an ethnic subgroup, which is a subsystem of a neighborhood system, and so on.

A mental disorder in the individual may be one manifestation in him of strain in some or all of these systems; and investigation with a broad focus will probably reveal a variety of other manifestations of strain, physical, psychosocial, and sociocultural, not only in him but in other individuals in the various groupings, and also in the patterns of energy and information transfer and boundary maintenance in the different systems.

Moreover, these disorders and signs of strain may stimulate remedial reactions in a variety of more or less organized and related caregiving and control systems of the community, such as those of health, mental health, welfare, education, corrections, manpower, religion, and law. Unfortunately, each of the caregiving systems is currently likely to identify only those signs of strain which are categorized as appropriate grist for its mill. Educators will define the problem as reading disorder in an underprivileged child; the police will define it as delinquency in a child who steals an automobile; the welfare worker as an A.D.C. problem in an unmarried woman who is a newcomer to the city and has three children; the city hospital, as a medical problem of a woman with high blood pressure who has to care for three children.

The ecological systems model attempts to bring all these factors into mutual articulation. It points to the design of a comprehensive system of caregiving units and an attempt to orient this to a broad view of the strains and maladjustments on a variety of levels of the client systems, subsystems, and individuals. What the implications of this model will be for future patterns of practice it is too soon to say. One possibility is a local Human Services Program, in which the various caregivers from the health, mental health, welfare, child and adult education, law, corrections, religion, and manpower facilities will be integrated and possibly housed in one neighborhood comprehensive community center, with more specialized larger district center staff on call or providing regional services on a scheduled basis.

Model of Shared Professional Domains

Concepts such as the catchment area and the Human Services Center will demand a new model of professional domains to replace the traditional model of contiguous nonoverlapping domains, with referral of clients across the boundaries when they make contact with a professional or an agency whose specialized categorical program they do not fit.

The new model will emphasize the inevitability that many clients and problems can be handled just as effectively by alternative caregivers. Each caregiver will abstract from the multifactorial predicament of the client certain aspects, to which his professional training and experience have sensitized him, and for the handling of which he has specialized skills. Because there are many factors involved, it is conceivable that a number of different interventions may result in swinging the balance of forces in a desirable direction.

Professionals, according to this new model, must be trained to recognize that their's is only one of a variety of possible approaches, and that other specialists can make a valid alternative contribution to a particular case. They must learn to realize that they can make a generalist as well as a specialist contribution to any case, and also to accept and value a commitment to give generalist guidance and supervision to a wide range of cases. Wasteful referral of "unsuitable" cases to other agencies will then be much reduced, and will be replaced by involving other specialists in collaborating on shared cases. Also, professionals will be trained to try and attract other professionals and nonprofessionals to help them, and to bring them in to share their domain, instead of marking out the boundaries of the domain and then fighting off potential intruders.

Index

Abortion, 56, 98, 106, 107, 150-1, 199, 252

Action for Mental Health, 188

Adjusting Overseas, 214

administrative action, 43

adolescence xv, 10, 36, 76, 207, 213

aged, xv, 17, 197-8, 200, 246, 252

Alaska, 187

Alcoholics Anonymous, 20, 224

alcoholism, 20, 21, 199

alienation, 36, 190, 247

American Association of Retired Persons, 18

amputees, 22, 83

anti-poverty movement, 222

appendicitis, 219

Arab-Israeli War, 1967, 167, 168

Arabs, 166, 172

army officers, 87

associations and groups, 5, 6, 16-25, 34, 142, 224-5, 229-30

balance of forces see: equilibrium and disequilibrium

bartenders, 12, 210-11

bedwetting, 67, 68

bereavement, xiv, 14, 15, 22, 56-8, 80, 107, 151-5, 202, 204-5

birth defects, 14, 49, 50, 57, 155, 204

Bishop-to-Bishop Coordinate Status Committee, 28

Black Death, 19

blacks see: minorities

blood pressure, high, 254

Boston, 33, 34, 35, 45, 56, 187, 210

Boston Lying-In Hospital, 48

259